bones

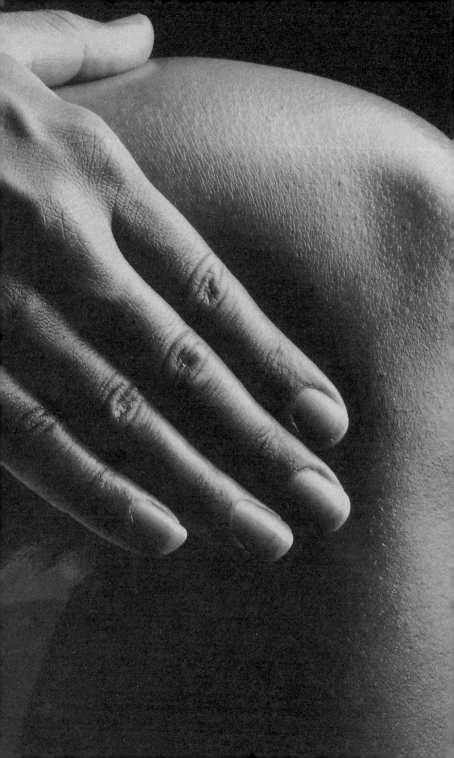

bones

your 100 questions answered

Dr. Caroline Shreeve

Newleaf

First published by

NEWLEAF

an imprint of

GILL & MACMILLAN LTD

Hume Avenue, Park West, Dublin 12

with associated companies throughout the world

www.gillmacmillan.ie

ISBN 0 7171 3265 X

A CIP catalogue record for this book is available from the British Library.

Note from the publisher
Information given in this book is not intended to be
taken as a replacement for medical advice. Any person with
a condition requiring medical attention should consult a
qualified medical practitioner or therapist.

This book was conceived, designed and produced by

THE IVY PRESS LIMITED

ART DIRECTOR Peter Bridgewater
PUBLISHER Sophie Collins
EDITORIAL DIRECTOR Steve Luck
DESIGNER Jane Lanaway
PROJECT EDITOR Georga Godwin
DTP DESIGNER Chris Lanaway
MEDICAL ILLUSTRATOR Michael Courtney

Printed in Spain by Graficomo, S.A.

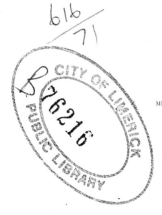

Contents

Introduction

To many of us bone problems mainly mean fractures, sprains and dislocated joints, diagnosed on X-ray and cured by immobilization (such as a splint), exercise or rest. Congenital (birth) deformities and metabolic disorders of the skeleton, inflammation and infection, secondary cancerous deposits, and benign and malignant bony tumours spring less readily to mind. Yet bones are susceptible to many of the diseases afflicting the rest of the body, as well as to others peculiar to themselves.

Despite its appearance, bone is far from inert. Arteries supply it with oxygen-rich blood and nutrients, while veins drain the used blood away to recycle it through the heart, kidneys and lungs. Lymph vessels provide lymph, which is rich in white blood (defence) cells, before removing it for the immune system to replenish. Nerves supply bones with pain, temperature and other sensations and, in the long limb bones especially, a constant cycle of destruction and rejuvenation removes bone eroded by stress, age or illness, replacing it with new.

Lifestyle, age and family traits all affect the skeleton's composition. Our bones grow and strengthen until our teens or twenties, provided that we exercise, have sufficient exposure to sunlight and eat an adequate diet. They remain at their healthiest for the next ten years, compensating for any loss of calcium and phosphate into the bloodstream by efficient resorption and assimilation. From our early thirties onwards, however, our bones start to develop a mineral deficit. They lose calcium and phosphate, and become less competent at replacing them. This sets the scene for brittle bone disease (osteoporosis), a condition affecting three to five per cent of post-menopausal women and a significant number of older men.

Good Health: Bones – Your 100 questions answered includes several questions and answers on osteoporosis, a major cause of serious (often life-threatening) fractures from middle age onwards. The complications of a fractured neck of the femur (thigh bone), for example – shock, fat embolism and increased accident-proneness – claim many lives, and its prevention is one of the main aims of prescribing (and taking) hormone replacement therapy (HRT). This book also covers other metabolic bone disorders, such as infantile rickets and Paget's disease.

One advantage of our growing acceptance of complementary medicine is an increased awareness of the importance of preventative measures. Governments are suitably attuned, for instance, to

Skull
Orbit
Mandible
Vertebral column
Clavicle
Scapula
Sternum
Humerus
Ulna
Radius
Carpals
Metacarpal
Phalanges
Sacrum
Rib cage
Tibia
Pelvis
Femur
Datella
Fibula
Tarsals
Metatarsals
Phalanges

There are roughly 206 bones in a skeleton that work together to support and protect the internal organs.

the emphasis of the National Heart Foundation and the World Health Organization (WHO) on regular exercise and a broad-based low-fat diet to minimize the risks of cardiovascular disease, heart attacks and strokes. Dietary and exercise advice are now similarly available for the maintenance of healthy bones, following controlled studies in the US and Europe of several related factors. Running and jumping activity in pre-pubertal children; the effect of sunlight (or its lack) upon the manufacture of vitamin D by the skin; the RDAs (recommended daily allowances) of calcium, phosphate, magnesium and other salient nutrients; and the need for multivitamin, mineral and calcium supplements – all these have come under review.

In fact the growth of 'other' medical wisdom nurtured by our New Millennium urge for a more rounded health philosophy has taken preventative medicine a step closer to the holistic viewpoint. It is becoming increasingly clear that lifestyle changes contribute more than risk reduction for serious disorders. Their advocates are discovering increased energy and vitality, improved physical and mental function and an enhanced definition of our tripartite nature of body, mind and soul.

Foods for healthy bones (such as reduced-fat milk, cheese and other dairy products, green leafy vegetables and protein foods, rich in calcium, magnesium, amino acids and trace elements) also promote calmness, improved sleep and a healthy nervous system. Exercises to encourage bone renewal, strengthen the spine and muscles, tendons and ligaments can also release mood-improving endorphins and the neurotransmitter serotonin. Active in promoting a sense of well being and sounder sleep, this chemical messenger produced by the brain also raises the pain threshold, blunting our perception of painful stimuli – an especially important benefit to sufferers from arthritis, spondylitis, sciatica and other chronic conditions.

Good Health: Bones – Your 100 questions answered is compiled from the many questions that patients ask their doctor, puzzle or worry over, look up in medical encyclopaedias or on the Internet and/or discuss with family and friends. The answers are as detailed as space allows, while steering clear of unnecessary technicalities and explaining those that need to be included.

The first part of this book ('Prevention') deals with general bone health and maintenance. It touches on a number of disorders which are dealt with more fully in the second part and provides information on such diverse topics as the 'funny bone', whether men have fewer ribs than women, whether 'breaking every bone in your body' can literally be true and why the bones in our feet do not wear out. It also explains fractures: how long they take to heal and how bones mend, why some babies are born with squashed-looking heads and how bones grow – and know when to stop growing.

The second part of the book ('When things go wrong') deals with the main injuries to, and disorders of, the skeleton. This part is divided into sections arranged according to body parts. It answers general questions about skeletal disorders, such as fragile bone disease (an hereditary complaint affecting infants and children, unrelated to brittle bone disease or osteoporosis), achondroplasia (stunted growth), bone-density heel scans and secondary cancer deposits in bone. This part also deals with the cervical (neck) vertebrae, including the mechanism by which injuries and dislocations in this region can cause head, neck, shoulder and upper limb pain extending to the fingertips. It looks at the unusual symptoms that an extra (cervical) rib can cause; explains why a metal plate is sometimes inserted into the skull; examines the causes and consequences of orbital (eye orbit) fracture; and discusses infection of a neck bone mimicking meningitis. The 'When things go wrong' part also explains the causes of chronic spinal pain and abnormal spinal curvature and examines some of the treatments. This is followed by sections on ailments that affect the limbs, and finally a section on the various different treatments that may be offered to you, from gold injections for rheumatoid arthritis to hydrocortisone for a painful shoulder, and a discussion of the merits – or otherwise – of complementary treatments.

Prevention

This section provides basic information about your bones: what they are made of and how they function. It answers questions about keeping your bones healthy and how to recognize the first signs that something may be wrong. It also offers useful background knowledge about many of the less serious ailments, especially fractures, and the kinds of treatment you can expect.

I am 38 and the single mother of two small children. I feel so stiff and sore first thing in the morning, just when I need all my energy. Should I see my doctor?

There are several reasons for morning stiffness, including poor sleep. Both mind and body need complete relaxation in order to maximize the repair of daily wear and tear in muscles and joints. Waking several times during the night, or tossing and turning, can leave you aching all over. Your nights are bound to be disturbed sometimes by your children and if your children are poor sleepers, then your doctor may be able to offer advice.

You may drop off to sleep the moment you hit the sheets, but your joints remain tense unless your mattress firmly supports your entire spine. A suitable pillow is equally important – ones that are too hard or too high can give you a crick in the neck, while soft ones support your head at an incorrect angle. You can prepare your mind, muscles and joints for a night's healthful rest by having a long, warm shower or bath using the aromatherapy oils calamine or rosemary. Calamine herbal tea before bed is also soothing, as is a milky drink, since the calcium aids the relaxation of muscles, which in turn eases the joints. Check your posture. A manual job usually works the spine and main limb muscles, whereas in the office long intervals seated on a hard chair, often of unsuitable height, working at a computer with a mouse-pad in an awkward place can cause shoulder and wrist strain. ●

2 My sister was born
with an odd-shaped
head, but now, at the
age of three months,
it looks quite normal.
Can you explain this?

Your sister's head was an odd shape when she
was born because of a process called moulding,
which took place as she passed through your
mother's birth canal as she was being born. Moulding
makes it possible for a baby to fit through the
opening in the lower part of the hipbone. Sometimes
surgical forceps are needed to pull the head down
and aid delivery, which can leave an infant's head
bruised and temporarily misshapen.

The baby's skull has 22 bones which interlock
with one another along edges (or sutures) notched
with minute, wavy lines. Connective tissue (the
sutural ligament) cements these together. Especially
prominent in babies and young children, this tissue
allows for a certain amount of 'give', or conformity,
to take place when external pressure is applied.

The skull bones are irregular plate-shaped
structures, more elastic in infants than in adults. At
birth the bones on the top and sides of the cranium
are separated from each other by webs of boneless
membrane (the so-called 'soft spots'). There are two
such spaces (or fontanelles) on top of the head – a
lozenge-shaped one in front and a smaller, triangular
one behind. These fontanelles also contribute to the
plastic quality of a newborn infant's skull and to the
moulding process but it is not these which made
your sister's head an odd shape. ●

3 Bones look completely solid, so how do they grow? And what makes them stop growing?

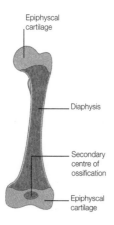

Epiphyscal cartilage

Diaphysis

Secondary centre of ossification

Epiphyscal cartilage

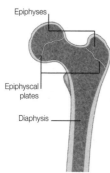

Epiphyses

Epiphyscal plates

Diaphysis

The femur is a typical long bone, with a shaft (diaphysis) and ends (epiphyses) which help to form the hip joint above and the knee joint below.

Bones look solid, but they are composed of living tissue and are supplied with arteries, veins and nerves. Their interiors are hives of metabolic industry covered by an opaque white surface.

The main shaft of the femur, for example, has ends covered with cartilage for smooth movement in the hip and knee joints. The rest of the bone is covered with a thin membrane (periosteum) that adheres to its surface. Near the centre of the shaft a small opening transmits an artery, veins, nerves and lymphatics into the bone's interior. There are similar smaller holes at the bone's extremities.

Cutting the femur lengthways reveals an outer shell of hard compact bone (the cortex) and a central cavity (the medulla), which is filled with red bone marrow before puberty and yellow marrow – mainly fat – thereafter.

Bones grow both lengthways from the clear white line of cartilage at each extremity and width wise by laying down new bone beneath the periosteum. Several hormones stimulate and control bone growth. Growth hormone from the pituitary gland in the brain stimulates epiphyseal growth, while sex hormones prompt the growth plates to mature and close, bringing growth to an end. Disruption of the balance between these two can cause problems in the development of the skeleton. ●

4 My five-year-old daughter is a real tomboy but, despite numerous falls, she has never broken any bones. Can you explain this?

Children's bones are springy and more resilient than those of an adult. Although they can snap right through, they more often bend and buckle. Such 'greenstick' fractures can easily be overlooked, because the usual fracture signs may be absent. Youngsters of your daughter's age can injure themselves more seriously than is at first apparent. Frequent fracture sites in children include the collar bone, the lower leg above the ankle and both ends of the humerus (upper arm bone).

Stunted growth and deformity are the chief dangers caused by undiagnosed fractures. The cartilaginous growth plates (*see Q 3*) at the ends of the long bones are especially vulnerable. And certain kinds of trauma can wrench off the bone's upper or lower end so a bony bridge can form leading to premature fusion. If fusion becomes complete, all growth ceases at that point. If it is partial, growth ceases at the fused area but persists in the adjacent undamaged areas, causing an angulation deformity.

If a fracture causes the growth to stop in one bone of a pair, such as the forearm or lower leg, the deformity which follows is dramatic. Treatment is often required for the prevention or correction of such damage. The safe approach is to consult a doctor and ask for x-rays of any injury in a young child that looks the slightest bit suspicious. ●

Greenstick fracture

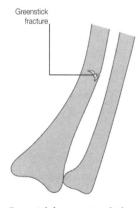

Greenstick fractures, in which the bone splits but does not break completely through are usually more common in children than adults.

5 **How long do bones take to mend after being broken?**

The length of time that bones take to repair themselves depends upon a person's age and state of health, whether the broken fragments are out of alignment (displaced), where they occur and whether the injury has disrupted the blood supply.

Children's fractures generally heal quickly, once they have been diagnosed. Fractures in babies may be securely united in two to three weeks. After growth stops (see Q 3), age ceases to be a factor, although the bones of both sexes start to lose 'mass' (substance) from around 30 years onwards.

Health factors that influence bone repair include inherited metabolic weaknesses, poor nutrition and osteoporosis (see Q 26).

Bones that are slightly out of alignment can heal by producing bony repair material without the fracture having to be realigned before setting (reduced) while significant misalignment needs to be reduced and the part immobilized with a plaster cast to prevent pain and deformity and some bones are prone to blood-supply problems (see Q 79).

Simple fractures heal more readily than compound fractures where the damaged bone and the body's surface connect and infections can hamper healing. 'Comminuted' fractures, in which bones are broken into more than two fragments, also take longer to heal. ●

Callus

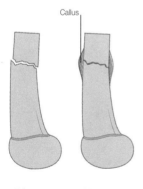

All fractures start to heal straightaway. Generally, the callus which protects the bone whilst it is healing can be seen by x-ray as early as two weeks after the break occured.

Why, in order to benefit bones, should exercise involve the feet striking a hard surface? Is bone strengthened and renewed like other body tissues?

Various theories have been put forward to explain how weight-bearing exercise specifically benefits the adult skeleton (*see Q 16*). The risks of non-weight-bearing exercise in young men were highlighted by astronauts, who were found to lose bone density after being in space. Prolonged bed-rest also leads to diminished bone mass.

The theory that brisk walking and jogging can 'drive calcium out of the bloodstream into the bones' is too simplistic. A paper in the *Lancet* in 1993 on the destruction and formation of bone tissues suggested that there is a continuous preventive maintenance programme by which adults replace old bone with new. This occurs at an annual rate of around 25 per cent in the bone's interior and at two to three per cent in the outer-layer. Remodelling takes place in areas probably stimulated by random triggers throughout the skeleton. The complete remodelling cycle takes several months, leaving small packets of bone in the interior, and new bone complete with its blood supply in the outer layer.

The factors that trigger remodelling are unclear, but changes generated by stress (such as weight-bearing exercise) are believed to play a part. Other factors, possibly hormonal, are thought to initiate the reversal phase, in which bone resorption ceases and is replaced by re-formation. ●

Q

7 Is it an old wives' tale that fish oil 'oils the joints'?

Many old wives' tales turn out to contain a grain of truth. Fish oil can benefit inflamed, painful joints, although it does not actually lubricate them. Some arthritis sufferers rub fish oil into their painful joints, but although a small quantity will be absorbed into the bloodstream, for effective relief the oil has to be taken by mouth.

Scientific interest in fish oils started in the mid 1970s when the Dutch investigators H. O. Bang and Jorn Dyerberg discovered that Greenland Eskimos, who eat a great deal of oily fish, have a low incidence of heart disease. The essential nutrients in fish oil that actively help the joints can be manufactured from the active ingredient in evening primrose oil, familiar to many women as a remedy for PMT, but the process is slow.

Fatty fish (such as tuna, sardines, mackerel, herring and salmon) are our richest source of the active nutrients in fish oil, which give rise to prostaglandins, which in turn play a vital role in the minute-by-minute regulation of cellular processes throughout the body and combat inflammation which occurs within the joints. Clinical studies in Europe have shown fish-oil extracts to be especially useful to rheumatoid arthritis sufferers, possibly because of an additional effect on the auto-immune response (*see Q 33*). ●

668 65

My cousin, aged ten, has won a scholarship to a ballet academy, and my aunt is terrified that she will ruin her feet. How can she minimize any damage?

Many mothers worry about the effects of ballet lessons on their daughters' feet, but it is usually only the very talented who practise long enough for injury to become a consideration. Potential damage is minimized by the use of a sprung floor. Feet are perfectly adapted to the attainment of truly staggering performances, if the movements are practised safely (*see Q 19*).

Stress fractures (*see Q 71*) are not an issue for young children, whose bones are tougher and less brittle than an adult's. Activity helps develop their leg muscles, which grow firm and strong. Very young children rarely attend classes for more than half an hour twice weekly, and the aim is to nurture flexibility rather than physical strength. They do not start pointe-work (dancing on the points of the toes) until they are ready, which varies from 11 to 15.

Regular footwork exercises are used to maintain suppleness, with warming-up and cooling-down a priority. The correct footwear is vital which also helps maintain optimal circulation in the feet to reduce the risks of muscle strains and cramps.

Regular exercise is also desirable to maintain overall physical agility and co-ordination. And a balanced diet aids growth, development and stamina. Herb bath additives can soothe tired feet and bruises respond well to homeopathic ointments. ●

9 **Can a dislocated shoulder joint be strengthened to prevent it slipping out of place in future?**

Surgery is usually needed to strengthen a shoulder that continues to 'slip out of place'. The shoulder is a ball-and-socket joint formed by the spherical upper end of the upper arm bone, fitting into the shallow, saucer-shaped cavity on the side of the scapula (shoulder blade). Dislocation generally involves the upper arm bone slipping forwards (anterior dislocation) out of its normal position.

Backward (posterior) dislocation can occur by rotating the shoulder violently inwards. Anterior dislocations are especially painful but, in both cases, the shoulder becomes misshapen. Following an x-ray to confirm the position of the displaced bones, the dislocation is reduced as soon as possible under a general anaesthetic.

Recurrent dislocations can result from the torn membrane failing to heal after being stripped from the rim of the joint cavity, or from damage to the surface of the head of the humerus. Surgery prevents further dislocation by repairing the torn tissues at the front of the joint. Voluntary partial of full dislocation can be treated by persuading patients to stop dislocating their own shoulder (as they tend to be able to do), or a bone graft (*see Q 17*) to enlarge and deepen the cavity. ●

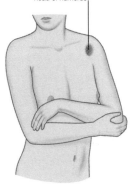

Hollow area due to the displacement of the head of humerus

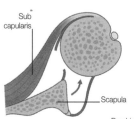

Sub capularis

Scapula

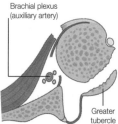

Brachial plexus (auxiliary artery)

Greater tubercle

An anterior dislocation is rare in children but is a common injury in the 18–25 age group (largely due to sport), and in the elderly.

Q

My nine-year-old daughter was recently diagnosed with asthma, and our doctor wants to prescribe a steroid inhaler. I have heard that this can stunt a child's growth. What is your opinion?

It has been known for some time that children treated with inhaled steroids grow more slowly for a time, followed by a catch-up period. A Danish study looked at more than 200 children over a 15 year period. It found that the 142 children treated with inhaled budesonide eventually reached their normal height, although their growth rate slowed in the first year of using the drug. The average daily dose given to these children was the commonly prescribed 400 micrograms. The children were considered to have reached adult height when their growth rate at the age of 15 or over was less than 5mm (¼in) in two consecutive years. All the children reached their 'target' adult height (calculated from the height of their parents) to the same extent as healthy siblings. However, it is not yet known how other steroids, such as beclomethasone affects a child's growth.

Uncontrolled asthma has a more serious effect on children's growth than inhaled steroids, but the latter should still be used at the lowest dose. Many doctors monitor children's growth while they are under treatment, and the effects on their bone density also need to be considered. Adequate supplies of calcium are essential, and a daily calcium supplement is a wise precaution, especially for children on higher doses of inhaled steroids.

11 **How many bones do we have in our bodies? Can the expression 'broke every bone in his body' literally be true?**

The number of bones in the adult human skeleton depends on whether certain bones are included in the total: 200 is a commonly agreed figure, including 26 in the spine, eight in the cranium, 14 in the face, 64 in the upper limbs and 62 in the lower limbs. The sternum (breastbone), the ribs and the hyoid bone, which supports the tongue, account for the remaining 26. This system includes the kneecaps, but excludes bones that develop inside tendons, and the three bones of the middle ear.

Various classification systems for bones have been devised, with one of the simplest depending on the shape of the bones. Long bones are found in the limbs, where they act with the great muscle groups, keeping the body erect and effecting movement. Also the collar bone and bones in the feet and hands. Short bones are found in the wrists and ankles and tend to be sturdy, bound together by ligaments. Flat bones include the shoulder blades and the skull. The final group of bones – irregular or mixed bones – stand in a class of their own because of their peculiar shape. Examples include the butterfly-shaped interior skull bone, the hyoid bone, the vertebrae and the coccyx (tailbone).

Nothing is impossible, but a person would be highly unlikely to break every bone in his body, unless he were literally crushed to death. ●

Q

12 **I've heard of ligament and cartilage damage to the knee. What exactly lies inside this joint?**

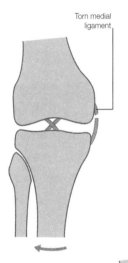

Torn medial ligament

Cruciate ligaments

Tearing the ligaments is a common sports injury. The patient can either tear just the medial ligament, or that and the cruciate ligaments.

The knee is formed by the lower end of the thigh bone and the upper end of the shin bone on the one hand, and by the lower end of the thigh and the kneecap, (*see Q 73*) on the other. It is almost entirely enclosed by a tough fibrous membrane strengthened by ligaments. Crescent-shaped cartilages and cross-shaped ligaments within the knee promote the joint's complex movements.

Overextension of the knee is prevented, and stabilization of the knee in a fully straightened position created, by means of two ligaments. Rupture of either or both of these leaves the lower leg dangling uselessly.

The two crescent-shaped cartilages are attached to the upper surface of the shin bone. They naturally move with the shin, but part of the inner (medial) cartilage is also attached to the thigh bone and must move with it. Because this is more firmly fixed, it is torn around eight times as often as the outer cartilage. This is usually a football injury, but is also common among people who work in a squatting position. Besides their role in the knee's movements, the crescent-shaped cartilages are also concerned with its lubrication, acting like sponges in absorbing the synovial fluid.

13 **How can you tell where poor posture ends and spinal disorders begin?**

It can be difficult to distinguish between the two – it is often only a matter of degree. The normal upper back is convex, and many people slouch and have round shoulders, but kyphosis (exaggeration of the spinal curve) is diagnosed only when that curve is excessive. The normal neck and lower back are concave: a reversal in this shape is called kyphosis; possible causes include a compression fracture (*see Q 26*) and ankylosing spondylitis (*see Q 47*).

Lordosis is the opposite of kyphosis – instead of round shoulders, the person has an excessively hollow back. Poor posture is nearly always to blame, although it is occasionally seen counterbalancing kyphosis above or below, or a deformity of a hip joint. Scoliosis is lateral (sideways) curvature of the spine. The most important type – idiopathic structural scoliosis usually starts between 10–12 years old and continues until growth ceases. In the area of the curvature the vertebrae rotate, twisting their bodies towards, and their spinous processes away from, the curve. The outlook in cases of lumbar scoliosis is good, but thoracic scoliosis in a young child is more serious. Corrective surgery is generally deferred until early adolescence, to minimize height loss following fusion of the growing spine. In the meantime an orthotic brace may be prescribed to prevent further deterioration. ●

POOR POSTURE

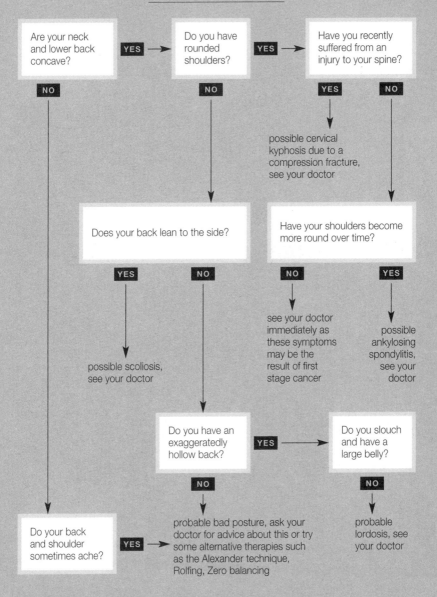

You should always consult your doctor when suffering from unexplained back pain.

Q

14 My husband is a fitness freak. Can overexercising damage his joints?

Overdoing any exercise can be damaging. Taxing aerobic exercise should probably not be performed for longer than 30 minutes more than three to four times a week by anyone over 25 without first consulting a doctor.

Your husband may be at increased risk of osteoarthritis – punishing exercise regimens are at least partly responsible for osteoarthritis, although lack of exercise is also a trigger. In most cases there are other predisposing factors, such as obesity, joint irregularities. Roughened or damaged joint interiors following rheumatoid arthritis, haemophilia joint damage or gout also readily become affected.

The articular cartilage in osteoarthritic joints gradually wears away, leaving the underlying bone exposed. Symptoms usually appear very gradually from middle age onwards, and people who exercise regularly may increase their activity in a bid to 'beat' the ageing process. However, this only further injures their joints. As their pain, stiffness and restricted movements worsen, some sufferers seek medical attention, although in many cases the discomfort never reaches that stage.

Seek medical advice for all injuries, and rest whenever this is advised. Qualified fitness experts can provide guidance on suitable exercises to suit a person's age, ability and health. ●

The saying 'don't take backache lying down' is all very well, but no one knows the agony I suffer from my back. Isn't this just an excuse from doctors who don't care?

Backache is one of the most common complaints about which patients consult their doctors. It is a symptom, not a disease, with possible causes running into thousands.

When you visit your doctor he may prescribe painkillers. If x-rays and tests are all normal, your doctor may refer you for physiotherapy, for which you may have to wait weeks. He may also recommend gentle exercise as many studies have challenged the notion that activity in backache sufferers should be restricted. A recent study in Boston found that intensive rehabilitation for patients with chronic low back pain increased significantly their physical activity level: 93 per cent of the 122 patients who completed a treatment programme were still performing stretches for the lower back and legs at least three times weekly 12 months later; 87 per cent were taking part in aerobic exercise three times weekly; 82 per cent were doing specific back-strengthening exercises; and 71 per cent were weight-training. The significant improvement in disability and pain after three months persisted at 12 months.

Specific disorders and injuries should of course be diagnosed and treated appropriately, but often, when no cause can be found, immobility simply aggravates rather than improves lower-back pain.

16 **Can lifestyle changes reduce the risk of fractures in older people?**

A healthy skeleton depends on an adequate calcium intake and regular exercise. Recent Canadian research studied 144 children aged eight to nine years with similar bone-mineral densities, 63 of whom played jumping games for 10–30 minutes three times a week, while the rest had regular physical-education classes. After eight months the first group had significantly higher bone-mineral density in the upper part of the thigh bone (where many fractures due to osteoporosis occur, *see Q 26*). Suitable exercises for an adult include skipping, dancing, walking and gentle jogging.

Dairy products are the richest source of calcium. Suggested amounts for women after the menopause range from 1,000 to 2000mg. A daily calcium supplement ensures that your requirement are met.

Other lifestyle factors which should be avioded include smoking and drinking large quantities of carbonated cola-type beverages which have recently been linked with an increased fracture risk in physically active teenage girls.

'Bumper bars' can reduce fractures from falls among the elderly by up to 50 per cent. Made of 1.5cm (½in) sheets of PVC plastic and foam, these are inserted into the pockets of tailor-made underpants: wearers then 'hit and roll' or bounce when they fall over, rather than 'hit and break'. ●

My best friend broke her leg badly, and it became infected and didn't heal. Now she is going to have a bone graft. Could you explain what this involves, and whether it will hurt?

B one grafts are used to help heal fractures, to fill a bone cavity and in an operation which fuses a joint (for instance, to control osteoarthritis).

Ideally bone grafts are obtained from another part of the patient's body to avoid rejection of the transplanted tissue. Bone tissue from another person can also be used. Animal bone (xenograft), mainly bovine, can also be grafted but is inferior to the patient's own bone graft and cannot be relied upon to become integrated into the new bone site.

Most of the transferred bone cells die, and the purpose of the graft is to provide a suitable scaffold upon which new bone will grow. The entire graft is ultimately replaced by the patient's new, living bone. The better the blood supply to the graft site, the better the chances of the new bone 'taking'.

Modern grafting techniques have a high success rate, because it is now possible to transfer bone with its soft-tissue coverings and a short stalk of blood vessels attached. These nutrient vessels are immediately joined up to corresponding ones in the new site, and the living graft rapidly becomes incorporated into the patient's tissues.

The operation planned for your friend will be performed under a general anaesthetic. She will feel sore when she wakes up, but hopefully the procedure will heal her fracture satisfactorily. ●

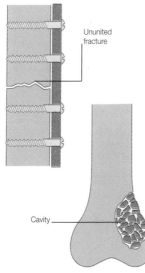

Ununited fracture

Cavity

Examples of two types of bone graft. ABOVE LEFT *A cortical slab graft held to the bone by pins.* ABOVE RIGHT *Cancellous grafts used to fill a cavity by the head of the bone.*

18 I am a boy aged 17. My best mate died six months ago of a cancer near his knee joint. Now I'm afraid of every little bump on my legs. What can I do to keep my bones cancer-free?

Osteosarcoma, the most likely tumour for your friend to have suffered from, typically affects children and young adults below the age of 20. It develops from primitive bone-forming cells, usually at the lower end of the thigh bone, the upper end of the main shin bone or upper end of the upper arm bone. The part where the tumour grows may feel hard and hot, and be swollen.

Osteosarcoma is highly malignant, forming secondary cancer deposits elsewhere in the body, often in the lungs. However, advances using intensive drug treatment in addition to surgery have now improved the recovery rate. Chemotherapy, which has major side-effects is usually started before surgery and continued at intervals for up to a year afterwards. It helps prevent the cancer from recurring, and from spreading elsewhere.

Nothing can guarantee you immunity from cancer, but you can reduce the risks. Ask your doctor to check any unexplained lumps or swellings. Follow the advice given for healthy bones (*see Q 16*). Prolonged stress, pollution (including smoking), ultraviolet light, viral infections and ageing all increase the body's free-radical production so eat a balanced diet: six to seven daily portions of fresh fruit and vegetables, milk and dairy products, meat, fish and eggs, grains and nuts. ●

Q

How are all the bones attached to one another in the foot, and why don't they wear out?

The foot consists of three groups of bones. The first of these (the tarsus) includes seven bones, one of which together with the lower ends of the two shin bones form the ankle joint (see Q 70). The largest tarsal bone (and biggest in the foot) is the calcaneum which is situated in the lower and back part of the foot and forms the heel. It transmits the weight of the body to the ground, forming a strong lever for the calf muscles.

The second group consists of the five metatarsals – the long bones of the foot that join the tarsals at their near end and the toe bones at their far end. Strong ligaments bind the foot bones together, including one called the spring ligament, which is primarily concerned with supporting the arch of the foot. Damage to this ligament leads to the condition of 'flat foot' (see Q 99).

The foot's third group of bones is comprised of 14 tiny 'long' bones: two in the big toe and three apiece in the remaining four toes.

The bones of the foot bear severe pressure and take the strain from the body's weight. They are protected from 'wearing out' by the rich supply of nutrient-bearing blood that is transported to them via the arteries. These enable the bone to renew itself as required, and to dispose of worn-out bone cells when necessary (see Q 6).

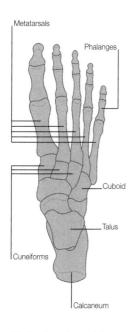

Metatarsals
Phalanges
Cuboid
Talus
Cuneiforms
Calcaneum

The foot is made up of three types of bones: the tarsals; the metarsals and phalanges, which includes the cuneiforms and calcaneum.

20 **Is it true that men have one fewer rib than women, and how do the ribs move when we breathe?**

Men and women both have 12 pairs of ribs, each adapted to its function and position. Together they provide a protective cage around the organs in the chest and they help the chest wall to expand and contract during respiration.

All 12 pairs of ribs are jointed to the thoracic vertebrae (upper spinal bones) and the upper seven pairs also articulate directly with the sternum (breastbone) in front. Rotating at the head end next to the spine; they move upwards and outwards as we inhale, downwards and outwards as we exhale, in synchrony with the diaphragm, which orchestrates our breathing. The upper seven pairs are termed 'true' ribs; the remaining five pairs, which are not attached directly to the sternum, 'false' ribs. Of these, the lower two pairs, which are shorter and end in free extremities, are known as 'floating' ribs.

A typical rib is twisted and bent forwards at an angle. It is attached by a ligament to a disk in the spinal column and moves with the corresponding vertebra. A groove running along the ribshaft's underside harbours the nerve, artery and vein supplying the rib and the intercostal muscles. The upper two pairs of ribs are stabilized and helped to rise by muscles coming from the lower cervical (neck) vertebrae. The lower ribs give rise to all the muscles that form the abdominal wall. ●

When things go wrong

This part of the book discusses the injuries and diseases common to the bones. It takes each part of the skeleton separately, explaining the causes of ailments and pain, and looks at the treatment options, in both orthodox and complementary medicine.

General questions

This section answers some of the most frequently asked questions about general disorders that can affect your bones. As well as looking at some of the more common problems, it also examines less well-known diseases, including those bone disorders that are a side-effect of other ailments.

21 I read a magazine article about a little girl of three whose bones broke at the slightest touch. Could you explain this disorder?

The disorder to which the article referred is fragile bone disease (fragilitas ossium). Present from birth and inherited in all but the most severe cases, it is caused by a defect in the formation of collagen, the tough connective tissue found throughout the skeleton and in skin, teeth, tendons and ligaments. The sufferer's bones are soft, brittle and fragile, breaking spontaneously or after the most trivial injury.

Babies with the worst form of fragile bones are born with multiple fractures and do not survive. Other children suffer fractures from birth onwards, often as many as 50 during the first years of life. Usually these quickly repair themselves (*see Q 5*), but the risk of deformity is high, from misalignment or from bending of the bones.

Some people with this complaint also suffer from otosclerosis, a disease of the middle ear in which the three tiny, usually mobile bones thicken and grow into one another, causing a form of hearing disability called conduction deafness. Lax ligaments are another common feature, compounding the already severe skeletal problems. A distinct blue tinge to the whites of the eyes may be present.

There is no cure for the underlying defect of fragile bones, but the fractures are generally treated like those of normal children. Major fractures of the long bones, such as the femur, are however sometimes repaired by internal fixation, to help minimize deformity and encourage an early return to normal activity. Walking calipers and other protective appliances are often of use to older children and adults.

Fragile bone disease is usually transmitted by a dominant gene in one or other parent. In one of the harshest forms, however, neither parent is affected, and the cause is thought to be either a fresh gene mutation or the combination of a recessive defective gene from each parent.

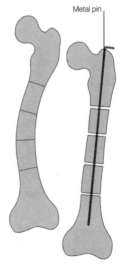

Metal pin

Fragile bones break easily and become bent and deformed. If this is very severe the child may become unable to walk and a metal pin is inserted to straighten the bone.

A cousin of my father suffered from stunted growth. Was this caused by his mother's diet during pregnancy, and can it be passed on?

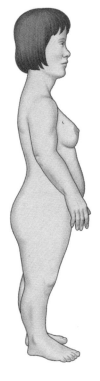

Achondroplasia means that whilst the torso grows to normal proportions the arms and legs are short.

Many conditions can cause stunted growth. Achondroplasia, the most common cause, affects about one in 25,000 children. The long bones of the limbs do not harden properly making the arms and legs very short.

Those affected tend to have large heads, the hands are small, and the feet short, flat and broad. The inlet of the hipbone is also affected which can lead to difficulties during pregnancy. Possible joint and bone problems include lumbar lordosis (*see Q 13*), bowed legs and an inability to straighten the elbows. Men reach an average height of about 132cm (52in), women of 122cm (48in). There is generally no intellectual impairment, and most people with this condition live as long as those of average stature.

Achondroplasia can usually be diagnosed at birth, although the large head may be mistaken for hydrocephalus ('water on the brain'), which does develop in some children; regular head measurements should be made to distinguish between the two. Changes in a single gene cause achondroplasia, which is in no way related to a woman's diet during pregnancy. Nine out of ten children with the condition are born to average-sized parents, but a couple with one average-statured and one achondroplastic spouse runs a 50 per cent chance of having an affected baby. ●

We are a professional Indian family. When our year-old son seemed unwell, we took him for a check and the doctor found that he had an enlarged head and swollen wrists and ankles. Tests revealed rickets, but isn't that a disease of the past?

Rickets, which was common in developed countries until the twentieth century, is caused by a deficiency of vitamin D, and by inadequate exposure to sunlight, which aids the production of this vitamin. Dark-skinned children run an increased risk, because the skin pigment melanin blocks some of the effects of the sun's rays.

Vitamin D promotes the absorption of calcium and phosphorus during digestion so a deficiency leads to poor absorption of these minerals. The blood level of calcium is then maintained at the expense of the bones, stopping developing bones from becoming hard and causing a general loss of density in the skeleton which shows up in X-rays.

Nutritional rickets is most often seen in children around the age of one. They may seem unwell, have swollen wrists, bowed lower legs, an enlarged head and perhaps some chest deformity as well as changes in the shape of bone endings. Some children may experience seizures (due to their low calcium level) and a swollen 'soft spot' (fontanelle, see Q 2) suggestive of meningitis or other brain-related disorders. Blood tests show raised levels of parathyroid hormones. Treatment with vitamin D and calcium is usually all that is required to correct the deficiency, although an operation may be needed to correct severe bony deformity. ●

My husband consulted our doctor about pains in his stomach, arms and legs. Blood tests showed a high level of calcium, and x-rays revealed worn-out areas in his skeleton. The diagnosis was a non-cancerous tumour on his parathyroid gland. Please can you explain this?

The parathyroid glands – four pea-sized glands on the underside of the thyroid gland in the neck – secrete a hormone (PTH) which controls bone absorption. Your husband's condition, parathyroid osteodystrophy, is due to an benign tumour (adenoma) on one of these glands where it is secreting excessive amounts of PTH thus speeding up the absorption of bone.

Bones gradually become soft, cysts can develop in the long bones, and the high concentration of calcium in the urine can lead to the formation of kidney stones. The pancreas may become inflamed, or a duodenal ulcer may form. Other symptoms include depression, poor appetite, constipation, dehydration and high blood pressure.

Tests show a raised level of calcium in the blood and urine, and x-rays may reveal the loss of bone density throughout the entire skeleton.

Mild symptoms may not require treatment beyond careful monitoring, a six monthly review and a constant high fluid intake to prevent kidney stones, although in severe cases an operation to remove the tumour may be needed. ●

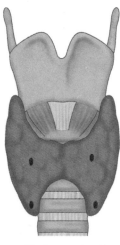

ABOVE The four parathyroid glands (shaded in red) are situated on the thyroid gland in the throat, RIGHT.

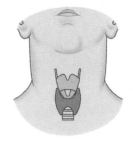

When my heel was checked in a pharmacy, the bone density was normal for my age (45). Does this mean that I will not need HRT?

Heel tests for bone density are done on many middle-aged women to check whether they are at risk of developing osteoporosis (brittle-bone disease, *see Q 26*). However, recent research, has shown that the bone density of the heel does not reflect bone-mineral density at the upper end of the thigh and in the spine, where most fractures occur. Heel tests of 1,000 women suggested that nearly 40 per cent of them had low bone densities, although only half had osteoporosis when tested using x-ray. And eight per cent of women with normal bone-mineral densities, according to heel scans, later turned out to have osteoporosis.

However, of the two-thirds of women over 65 tested, whom the test showed to have a low bone mass, 60 per cent had osteoporosis confirmed by x-ray. Heel scanning's most useful role is as a pre-screen test for post-menopausal women, ideally as part of an overall risk assessment that also considers other risk factors, such as family history, weight, smoking and past fractures. Women with positive results should then be reassessed using the more refined technique.

Whether or not to take HRT remains a dilemma for many, but its benefits are now known to extend beyond the skeleton to the brain, eyes, uterus (womb), skin and even mood.

26 Why do bones become fragile after the menopause, and does anything else weaken an adult's bones?

Strong, healthy bones have a high mineral content, but from around 30 years onwards they start to lose these minerals, becoming less resistant to falls and blows. At the menopause the ovaries stop secreting oestrogen, and the reduced level of this hormone accelerates the loss of calcium and phosphate beyond that of the natural ageing process. Bones losing density or 'mass' become porous and brittle, a condition known as osteoporosis or brittle bone disease. Consequences include fractures following minor accidents, the most common being the hip or a compression fracture of the spine, leading to the smallness of old people or a 'dowager's hump' between the shoulders.

Other factors that weaken adult bones include poor diet and a sedentary lifestyle. Diets low in dairy products increase the risk, while a lack of exercise increases the rate at which the skeleton loses minerals. An overactive thyroid gland, steroid drugs and prolonged bed-rest can also play a part.

Other diseases linked to osteoporosis include overactivity of the parathyroid glands (*see Q 24*) and primary biliary cirrhosis – a complaint of unexplained origin affecting the liver and gall bladder. Genetic factors play a part, as do smoking and drinking more than four alcoholic units a day for men, or three for women.

Our uncle, aged 55, is going very deaf and his head is enlarging – he has gone up two hat sizes in the past year. What is happening to him?

This sounds like Paget's disease one of the most common metabolic bone diseases. The affected skeletal area is broken down, then built back up, creating areas of high bone activity with an increased blood supply and soft, enlarged bones that fracture and deform. Any bone can be involved, but the most commonly affected are the hipbone, spine, shoulders and limbs. It can lead to dental problems, pressure on nerves in the skull causing deafness, headaches, fainting attacks and heart failure. Increased activity in bone development also raises the calcium level (*see Q 24*), causing kidney stones.

Inheritance plays a part in developing the disease, with 15–30 per cent of patients having other family members affected. Research also indicates that a 'slow' virus may be involved, (such as measles), although none has yet been identified.

All patients need lifelong monitoring, including input from an experienced orthopaedic surgeon. Paget's disease progresses along affected bones at a rate of about 1cm (½in) a year and does not jump joint spaces; but when it occurs on either side of a joint (especially a weight-bearing one), then severe osteoarthritis and deformity can result. Joint replacement is usually highly successful. Drugs to control the excessive resorption of bone are the mainstay of medical treatment. ●

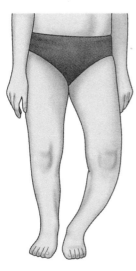

This illustration shows an example of the deformity caused by Paget's disease in the shin bone.

Q

28 **Our son, aged 15, is teased because he is 1.87m (6ft 2in) tall, but my husband and I are of medium height. Could something be wrong with him?**

Take your son to see a doctor if you are worried, but adolescent boys can grow to this height – and above – despite the height of their parents.

Perhaps you have been worried by stories of gigantism, a hormonal disorder in which children grow exceptionally tall? In this rare condition the long bones of the limbs become excessively long before growth ends (*see Q 3*). Gigantism is caused in the brain, which produces human growth hormone (HGH). Excessive amounts of HGH are released, while other symptoms can arise from pressure on the brain due to the tumour. Blood tests are taken to confirm the diagnosis, with the help of a skull X-ray and a scan to locate the tumour.

When a pituitary tumour produces large amounts of HGH in an adult, the condition is known as acromegaly. Adults remain the same height, but common changes include thickening of the facial bones, enlarged space between the teeth, increasing shoe size, and a deepening voice. Sweating and headaches, muscle weakness, and pins and needles in the hands are common. Similar symptoms may be present due to a brain tumour, and the same tests are largely used to diagnose the two conditions. Treatment involves surgery to remove the pituitary tumour, medication and radiation therapy. ●

My mother, who's 45, recovered from breast cancer, but now secondaries have been found in her bones. What exactly are they, and is there any cure?

Secondaries are tumours that have migrated through the body from their original site, such as the breast, and have developed in other areas. Secondary malignant tumours in bone are far more common than primary ones, and generally affect adults rather than children.

Tumours whose secondaries often appear in bone include tumours of the lung, prostate, thyroid gland, and the kidney. They tend to occur in the parts of the skeleton containing bone marrow: for example, the spine, ribs and hipbone, and the upper ends of the upper arm and thigh bones. They destroy the tissue supporting the marrow, replacing it with a tumour. Fractures due to diseased bone rather than injury are common, and along with pain are one of the first symptoms. X-rays show defined areas of destruction surrounded by unaffected bone. Osteoporosis (*see Q 26*) may be widespread, if secondaries have spread throughout the skeleton, and chest x-rays are normally taken to check for their presence in lungs.

Hormone therapy is a common treatment for secondaries from breast or prostate cancer, and removal of the adrenal and pituitary glands may slow progress. Radiotherapy is used to control pain, and chemotherapy may help to destroy the secondary deposits. Surgery is no help in treatment here. ●

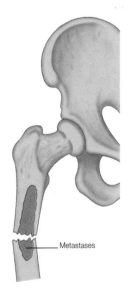

— Metastases

Secondaries of cancer (metastases) in the bones can lead to lack of bone density making them brittle and liable to break easily.

Q

30 Our son, aged seven, has a hard lump near his knee joint, which the surgeon thinks is non-cancerous. Could it still be dangerous, and are more swellings likely to appear?

This sounds like an osteochondroma, a benign bone tumour that develops from the growing epiphyseal cartilage plate (*see Q 3*) – for instance, at the upper end of the tibia near the knee joint. It first comes to notice as a hard, clearly defined swelling close to its joint of origin, but as the bone lengthens, the tumour gets 'left behind', appearing to migrate along the shaft towards its centre.

X-rays show it growing out from its site like a mushroom, with a narrow, bony stalk and a cartilage-capped head. An osteochondroma will continue to enlarge until the child stops growing and, even after that, the knobble of cartilage often remains in place. It does not become cancerous, but should be removed if it causes pain or persists after the child reaches puberty.

Though usually single, numerous osteochondromas develop in the condition known as multiple hereditary exostoses, when nests of cells develop into up to 20 bony outgrowths next to a joint, just like the single variety. In severe cases the bone ceases to grow and deformity can result.

Symptoms are pain or pressure caused by the swelling lumps. Sometimes a tumour may undergo malignant change, therefore any outgrowth causing symptoms should be surgically removed (especially, any that shows signs of turning cancerous). ●

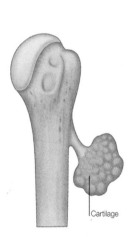

Cartilage

Osteochondroma which are non-cancerous tumours tend to grow out of the growth cartilage surrounding the bone and maintain a hard covering.

[44]

Q 31

Our father, who's 45, has been told that his painful toe is due to gout. How is this possible, since he's teetotal?

Alcohol is just one of a number of triggers of gout, which is a form of arthritis, 20 times more common in men than in women. Nearly all gout sufferers have an inborn defect in handling purine, a substance present in some foods. High levels of uric acid develop in the blood, leading to deposits of urate crystals in the joints, which become inflamed and their cartilage linings damaged.

Acute attacks can arise spontaneously, but may also follow injury, infection, unaccustomed exercise, starvation or the use of certain diuretic drugs. Typical sites include the big toe, finger and ankle joints, and the fibrous sac (bursa) at the point of the elbow. The affected area looks red, shiny and swollen, and feels hot and very painful. Attacks can become chronic, affecting other areas, with urate salts forming nodules (tophi) in tendons, bursae and cartilage, in and around joints and in the ear flap. Tophi often ulcerate, discharging a chalky substance, while the affected joints become increasingly stiff, painful and deformed. Urate crystals can form kidney stones, while micro-deposits throughout the kidneys' tissues may lead to renal failure.

Gout is generally diagnosed from a combination of the patient's symptoms and the presence of red shiny joints. X-rays show soft-tissue swelling and, occasionally, the asymmetrical punched-out bony 'cysts' that can develop in the bones. The diagnosis can be clinched by identification of the urate crystals in joint fluid.

Rest is essential during an acute attack of gout. Non-steroidal anti-inflammatory drugs (NSAIDs, *see Q 84*) will bring some relief. Gout- and uric acid-specific medications can be given at intervals if the attacks are frequent, and if tophi or kidney disease is present. You can help to counteract the effects of gout by avoiding foods rich in purine (offal, oily fish), obesity, heavy drinking and aspirin (which raises the blood uric-acid level).

Q

32 A deep cut on my husband's forearm seemed to heal. Then he became feverish, his wrist swelled and he was admitted to hospital. Is it something serious?

Your husband has septic arthritis – joint inflammation due to infection by bacteria carried to his wrist from the cut on his arm. Joints also become infected when bacteria on the skin reach the interior through a penetrating wound or from a nearby bone infection (osteomyelitis). The symptoms usually come on rapidly, but may take several days to develop. A feverish illness is typical, as are pain and swelling due to fluid escaping from the damaged tissues into and around the joint. The area may look red and feel warm to the touch, due to the increased blood supply. Pain limits movement, and in severe cases protective spasm in the adjoining muscles may prevent it altogether.

X-rays in the early stages usually appear normal, but a persistent joint infection damages the articular cartilage and sometimes the adjacent bone. Blood tests show an increased number of circulating white cells and other signs of inflammation. Bacteriological examination of fluid from the joint's interior will identify the responsible organism and its sensitivities to antibiotics.

Recovery from septic arthritis depends on the intensity of the infection and how the patient responds to treatment, which should be started promptly to eliminate or minimize permanent damage. The patient should rest in bed and take a suitable antibiotic until the bacteria's specific sensitivities are known. The joint is usually rested in a splint, and sustained traction may be applied to an infected hip or knee to relieve pain and muscle spasm. Joint fluid is aspirated (withdrawn) daily and replaced with a solution of the appropriate antibiotic until the patient's temperature returns to normal and the joint is no longer inflamed. Active movements are encouraged from then onwards, to restore the joint's function.

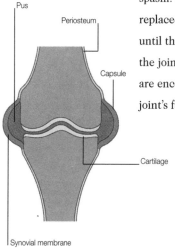

Pus

Periosteum

Capsule

Cartilage

Synovial membrane

When active, infective arthritis causes the joints to become distended as the capsulae fill with pus. The synovial membrane which normally protects the joint becomes inflamed and thickened.

My daughter, aged 35, has just been diagnosed with rheumatoid arthritis. How will it affect her?

Rheumatoid arthritis (RA) is an inflammatory disease producing pain, stiffness and swelling of the joints, usually in the hands, wrists, elbows, knees and feet. The illness generally starts between the ages of 25 and 50 and is three times more common in women. Symptoms develop with increasing pain and stiffness that is worse on becoming active after resting. It can affect the entire system with general feelings of sickness and fatigue, as well as weight loss and fever.

It is believed that RA is a condition in which the immune system attacks the person's own tissues. Viral or bacterial infection may also play a part. The membranes of affected joints become inflamed, and the underlying cartilage and bone around the joint become damaged. RA tends to grow less severe but joints are often permanently deformed.

Rest and a nutritional diet are important, especially during flare-ups. Non-steroidal anti-inflammatory drugs (NSAIDs) help to reduce inflammation and internal joint damage. Corticosteroid drugs reduce the effects during outbreaks. Injections of hydrocortisone into an affected joint can bring worthwhile relief, but there is some risk of accelerating the internal joint damage. Gold injections and cytotoxic drugs, which are toxic to human tissue, are still prescribed.

ARTHRITIS

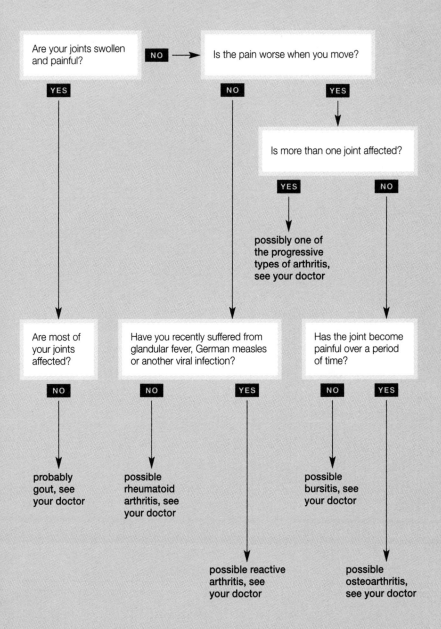

Are your joints swollen and painful?

NO → Is the pain worse when you move?

YES

NO

YES

Is more than one joint affected?

YES

NO

possibly one of the progressive types of arthritis, see your doctor

Are most of your joints affected?

NO

Have you recently suffered from glandular fever, German measles or another viral infection?

NO

YES

Has the joint become painful over a period of time?

NO

YES

probably gout, see your doctor

possible rheumatoid arthritis, see your doctor

possible bursitis, see your doctor

possible reactive arthritis, see your doctor

possible osteoarthritis, see your doctor

I damaged my left knee playing professional football as a lad. Now that I'm in my fifties it's becoming swollen and painful. My father had rheumatoid arthritis in his knees, so could I have the same ailment?

Your troublesome knee is most unlikely to be due to rheumatoid arthritis. RA (*see Q 33*), which nearly always starts before middle age, and it tends to affect several joints symmetrically. Your problem sounds like osteoarthritis (OA). You don't say whether your knee damage resulted from years of exercise and training or from a specific injury, such as a torn cartilage (*see Q12*), but both could increase the risks of degenerative joint changes as you grow older.

Here are further ways of distinguishing between the two types of arthritis: the pain of OA is aggravated by use and is worse (especially in weight-bearing joints) by the end of the day. RA pain is most severe when you move about after resting, and the joints are red, swollen and warm when the disease is active, whereas OA does not usually cause warmth and redness. OA joints tend to be stiff for brief periods; in RA, the stiffness is prolonged, especially in the morning. The muscles around your knee may cramp up to prevent you overusing it causing further damage. They would do the same around RA joints, but over time would cause deformity and loss of use. Being overweight aggravates either kind of arthritis, and many professional sportspeople put on weight when they cease training. Your doctor may prescribe anti-inflammatory drugs and/or physiotherapy. ●

I heard on the radio that they're using stinging nettles to treat osteoarthritis in Britain. Is there any value in this?

According to a report in the *Journal of the Royal Society of Medicine,* stinging nettles can relieve the pain and disability of osteoarthritis. The study involved 27 patients with OA pain at the base of the thumb or index finger, 19 of whom were taking simple analgesia (painkillers) and eight non-steroidal anti-inflammatory drugs (NSAIDs). All continued with their medication, but also used either stinging nettles or non-stinging dead nettles once daily for a week, rubbing the underside of the leaves onto the skin of the offending joints.

After a five-week break the groups reversed their treatment, recording levels of pain, disability and need for medication during each treatment phase. Reductions in the patients' scores for pain and disability were greater after using the stinging nettles than after the placebo treatment, and they also needed less medication. The greatest pain relief was experienced by the patients who developed weals. Eighty-five per cent of the patients found the stings an acceptable side-effect, and 50 per cent said they preferred using stinging nettles to their usual medication. Researchers at the University of Plymouth, who carried out the study, said that nettle sting contains serotonin, acetylcholine, histamine and leuktrienes which act upon nerve endings and may be responsible for the beneficial effects. ●

Head & neck

This section is relevant for two groups of people. First, for those who have never had any neck and upper back pain but hope to avoid it – a sensible course of action given the frequency with which such problems occur. The second group consists of those who have had problems with their head and neck before and hope to reduce the likelihood that they will have a further attack. It describes prevention rather than cure.

36 My neck and shoulders have been painful for months. My doctor called it 'degeneration' and prescribed painkillers, but isn't there any other treatment?

Most people over the age of 50 have some degeneration in the cervical (neck) vertebrae. Symptoms include a painful, stiff neck with tender neck muscles, a 'grating' sensation, shoulder and arm pain, and numbness and 'pins and needles' in the fingers. A tender scalp and nagging ache at the back of your head may also feature.

Sometimes the symptoms worsen for no apparent reason, but then retreat after weeks or even months of constant pain. In fact, they are almost always linked to and triggered by repetitive movements or strains. Typical examples of prime causes might be either sitting at a computer for hours wearing bifocal glasses, which force you to tilt your head back, or pushing your neck uncomfortably forward while lugging heavy shopping.

This condition – degenerative arthritis or cervical spondylosis – can result from injury, but is usually due to normal wear and tear; the lower three vertebrae just above shoulder level are most often affected. The discs between the vertebrae become thin, and the bone around their margins develop small bone spurs (osteophytes). The cartilages between the other, smaller joints also degenerate, producing osteoarthritic changes and more osteophytes. These then protrude into the spaces between the vertebrae, pressing on the cervical nerves. If the nipped tissues become inflamed and swollen, nerve-pressure symptoms then appear in the relevant areas.

Anti-inflammatory drugs, such as ibuprofen and naproxen, plus physiotherapy are usually prescribed to help reduce the inflammation and pain. Manipulation is sometimes recommended, but should be used with great caution by an experienced therapist because of the danger of osteophytes damaging the spinal cord. A close-fitting collar may be prescribed to rest and support the neck when symptoms are severe, and should be worn for one to three months, according to progress. ●

Q

37 **I'm a plumber, and I twisted my neck recently trying to reach a pipe. Two days later my neck got very stiff, and then the pain crept over my shoulder and down my right arm, and I'm now living on anti-inflammatories. What do you think this could be?**

You sound as though you might have a prolapsed disk in your neck. Typically the twisting strain that can give rise to this seems slight at the time and produces no discomfort until hours or even days later. The neck then becomes stiff and so painful that it is jarred by coughing, sneezing or some other minor strain. The pain usually extends over the shoulder and down the arm to the hand, and can cause tingling in the fingers.

The mechanical fault producing these symptoms starts with a tear in the fibrous capsule of the disk between the fifth and sixth, or the sixth and seventh, cervical vertebrae. Part of the disk's gelatinous filling ruptures through the tear, stretching a major pain-sensitive ligament and causing local pain in the neck. A larger protrusion pushes right through the ligament, where it can press on the adjacent nerve as it leaves the cervical spine, producing pain such as yours in the shoulder and arm. The worst-case scenario involves the errant jelly-like disk filling, impinging upon the spinal cord itself.

Mild to moderately severe prolapsed cervical discs tend to heal themselves, although the symptoms may take up to six months to disappear. Degeneration occurs more rapidly in a prolapsed disk, and osteoarthritis is likely to develop around it in the future. Treatment – if any – seeks to relieve pain and

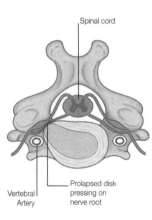

Spinal cord

Vertebral Artery

Prolapsed disk pressing on nerve root

Each vertebrae are separated by disks of cartilage which act like shock absorbers. When these 'slip' they press onto the spinal nerve causing pain.

restore normal function. Anti-inflammatory and pain-relieving drugs provide some relief, while a supportive collar may be prescribed to support the neck if symptoms are severe.

See your doctor without delay. A definitive diagnosis needs to be made in the case of all neck injuries, with a full assessment of the severity of the damage and the elimination of other causes. ●

Q

38 When my daughter, who's 24, went for a check-up, our doctor was puzzled because he could not feel a pulse in her left wrist. X-rays of her neck showed a cervical rib. What is this, and will it give her trouble later on?

A cervical rib is a hard fibrous outgrowth from part of a cervical vertebra on one or both sides of the neck. It can vary in size from a small bony knob to a complete extra rib, and while they rarely cause trouble during childhood, sagging of the shoulder with age can cause it to press on nerves or blood vessels, causing problems in the upper limb.

Symptoms usually appear around your daughter's age, and can best be understood from the viewpoint of the two major structures that arch over it, namely the main artery to the upper limb, and the lowest trunk or branch of the huge nerve complex running from the spinal cord to the upper limb.

The effects of pressure on these range from a dusky bluish colour in the forearm and hand to gangrene in the fingers. As in your daughter's case, the pulse at the wrist is often faint or absent. As well as numbness and pins and needles in the forearm and hand, especially along the inner (little finger) side; it is often relieved temporarily by changing the position of the arm. Effects on the muscles of the arms include weakness of the hand, with difficulty in carrying out finer movements.

Treatment depends on the severity of the symptoms and ranges from physiotherapy (shrugging exercises) in mild cases, to tone and lift the shoulder girdle, to removing the rib surgically. ●

Q

39 Following a whiplash injury, x-rays showed that I had dislocated a bone in my neck. I've been given a surgical collar, painkillers and an appointment to see a specialist in a month, but I'm in agony. Will he operate?

It sounds to me as though you have had a problem with your neck for some time. Whiplash trauma is unlikely, in itself, to 'sublux' (partially dislocate) a normal cervical vertebra forwards from its secure position on the one below it. Your present condition probably reflects a cervical instability somewhere in your past medical history. This sliding forwards (occasionally backwards) of a vertebra can occur gradually and spontaneously, but the severe overstretching (hyperextension) that your neck experienced when your car was hit probably made it happen again.

Possibilities range from past neck injury (presumably not in your case) through inflammation in the upper part of the neck (such as rheumatoid arthritis or a severe infection of the throat or gland) to a congenital defect. Symptoms include neck stiffness, pain and temporary deformity; and when inflammation is responsible (often in a child with an infected ear, throat or neck), the patient holds the head rigidly because the muscles are in spasm.

The most feared complication is damage to the spinal cord, but this is unlikely to happen to you because you have already been assessed and fitted with a suitable collar. Take your painkillers and seek medical attention if the pain remains severe. You are unlikely to undergo an operation if there is no sign of nerve damage: your progress may be assessed at regular intervals, or you may be advised to continue wearing the collar. If nerve damage does develop, then your affected vertebrae could be fused following skull traction, to reduce the dislocation. ●

40 I'm a 55-year-old woman, and although I've kept most of my teeth, my dentist said there was limited work he could do on the deep roots because my jawbone is soft. Is there any remedy?

There may be, but first you need a bone-densitometry scan, which your doctor can arrange for you.

We normally hear of the effects of osteoporosis on the upper end of the thigh bone, although brittle-bone disease also affects other skeletal areas, and the jawbone (and tooth loss) have been associated with it, as well as with increased periodontal disease (osteoporosis in the bones surrounding the teeth). Professor Elizabeth Krall of the Boston University Goldman School of Dental Medicine carried out a study to discover whether calcium and vitamin D supplements, taken to retard bone loss at the hip, would have a similar effect upon oral bone loss.

The study examined the pattern of tooth loss in 145 men and women aged 65 or older, over a five-year period. For the first three years the treatment group took 500mg/day of calcium and 700 IU (international units) of vitamin D, while the untreated group took placebo (dummy) tablets. All the volunteers had their teeth counted after six months and three years. The researchers took into account variables such as long-standing oral health, flossing, smoking and the use of water pills.

Members of the treatment group had a relative risk of tooth loss of much less than the placebo group, with 13 per cent losing teeth compared with 24 per cent in the untreated group. It was concluded that calcium and vitamin D supplements, increasingly recommended to prevent osteoporosis, 'could also end up saving a lot of teeth', in Professor Krall's words.

Q

41 My mother, aged 40, was knocked out with an iron bar. While she was in hospital a metal plate was inserted in her head. Won't it press on her brain, and will she ever have it removed?

It sounds as if your mother had a comminuted fracture of the skull, in which one of the large, plate-like bones of the skull broke into pieces. Because of the blow she received, her fracture was very likely also 'depressed', with bits of bone dented inwards (like the top of a boiled egg after being hit by a spoon). The injury area then becomes saucer-shaped, and the small bone fragments that form can cause irreversible damage to the soft tissue below.

The skull bones include the frontal bone, supporting the forehead and the front part of the top of the head; and the paired parietal bones, which meet on top of the head, in the skull's midline, and overlie brain lobes of the same name. These bones protect the sensory and motor regions of the brain, which control movement and sensation. Paired temporal bones protect the lower halves of the cerebral hemispheres, while the single occipital bone forms the back of the skull.

Three layers of membranes, called meninges also surround and protect the brain. Each of these varies according to their position in relation to the brain: the outermost membrane consists of tough fibrous tissue; the middle layer is thin and transparent and that closest to the brain, which follows every contour dipping in and out of every curve and furrow, is a tender layer. The brain is, therefore, well shielded by nature, but blows such as your mother received are obviously life-threatening. After repairing any tear in the meninges, the surgeon inserted a stainless-steel plate in the space vacated by the damaged skull bone, which he first removed. It will have been modelled to avoid pressing on the brain, but is vital to her welfare and will never be removed.

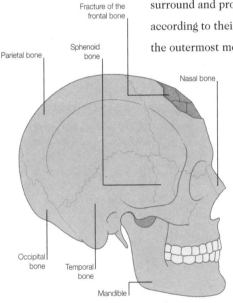

Fracture of the frontal bone

Parietal bone

Sphenoid bone

Nasal bone

Occipital bone

Temporal bone

Mandible

The skull is comprised of more than 20 bones. It is designed to protect the brain and so can take an amazing amount of pressure. However, knocks to the head can cause fractures.

Our neighbour's son, a policeman, was hit across the upper part of his face during an arrest, and he's now in hospital with a fractured orbit. What does this mean, and will he recover?

Your neighbour's son has fractured his eye socket which protects the eyeball from injury, and contains shock-absorbing fat, arteries, veins and nerves supplying the eyeball and its muscles. Most importantly, the optic nerve (which supplies sight) which passes through the socket as it attaches the eyeball to the brain.

The outlook depends on the severity and location of his fracture. Misalignment of broken fragments can have grave consequences, including brain damage. Disruption of the blood and nerve supplies to the eyeball can lead to partial paralysis of one or more of the muscles that move the eye in its orbit, thus affecting vision. Injury or severance of the optic nerve can cause partial or total loss of sight. You do not mention visual problems, so hopefully his injury is a small, hairline fracture that will soon heal.

Haemorrhage and infection are two possible complications of an orbital injury. An abscess in such a position requires urgent intervention by an ophthalmic surgeon, as does a build-up of blood from torn vessels. Teamwork involving ophthalmic and neurosurgical specialists might be required to deal with pus or blood escaping through a fracture at the rear of the orbit into the brain cavity. Meningitis and a brain abscess are just two of the possible problems that can arise.

43 My daughter, who is 19, was admitted to hospital with a fever, headache, stiff neck and difficulty in swallowing, but suspected meningitis turned out to be an infected bone in her neck. How did she get an illness like that?

An infection such as this can result from bacteria reaching the neck vertebrae in the bloodstream from a septic site elsewhere. Abscess formation, destruction of the affected vertebrae and adjoining disk, and pressure damage to the spinal cord are among the complications that can arise in the absence of prompt treatment.

Your daughter's fever, pain and difficulty in swallowing are typical symptoms. The condition is not always easy to distinguish from meningitis, or from tuberculosis of the cervical spine. The main pointers are the relatively rapid onset of the illness (compared with TB spine), the fever, swallowing problems and evidence of infection elsewhere.

Blood tests, and the identification of bacteria in pus drained from any abscess, clinch the diagnosis. Neck x-rays of someone who has suffered from the disease for days or weeks may show bone erosion, reduced disk space and possibly new bone formation underneath the cervical ligaments.

Treatment includes antibiotics; immobilization of the neck vertebrae in a plaster collar; and prompt drainage of any abscess, especially if there are signs of pressure upon the spinal cord, such as pain, weakness or tingling in the upper limb. The affected vertebrae usually fuse spontaneously as healing occurs, eliminating the need for surgical fusion.

Trunk & spine

This section answers frequently asked questions about disorders which affect the trunk and spine. Problems which affect this area of the skeleton are particularly worrying because by putting pressure on the spinal column they can have adverse affects throughout the body. The following answers give advice about prevention as well as cure, complementary as well as orthodox medicine.

44 My first pregnancy was terminated because the baby had spina bifida, but I don't understand this condition. Could it happen again?

Spina bifida literally means a 'spine divided down the middle'. The problem starts early in pregnancy, when the spinal tissues in the embryo fail to form a complete tube around the primitive spinal cord. As the baby grows, an opening develops in the spinal canal housing the spinal cord.

In its simplest forms, spina bifida occulta (meaning hidden) may produce no symptoms, with just one or more arches of the lumbo-sacral (lower back) vertebrae failing to meet in the midline. Occasionally the overlying skin may have a dimple, a tuft of hair, a fatty swelling (lipoma) or a sinus (a shallow tunnel connecting with deeper tissues). Affected babies may have some damage to the lower end of the spinal cord, with weak leg muscles, a limp, foot deformities (*see* Q 99) and/or urinary incontinence. A neurosurgical operation can sometimes help to prevent the condition worsening.

The more serious 'overt' form (spina bifida aperta) also involves the soft tissues and skin covering the spine, and sometimes the meningeal membranes enclosing the spinal cord. It can occur anywhere in the spine, but is most common in the middle of the back and causes varying degrees of muscular paralysis, as well as loss of sensation, bowel and bladder function. In the most serious form (rachischisis), the spinal cord is open and exposed on the surface, where it leaks fluid from its upper exposed part. In myelomeningocele there is no skin covering, and the spinal cord and nerve roots form a sac-like bulge on the outside of the body. In meningocele the bulging sac consists just of membranes and fluid, with normally situated nervous tissue. Many children born with myelomeningocele also have hydrocephalus ('water on the brain'), but do survive, due to treatment of the latter with a shunt – a tube draining excess cerebrospinal fluid from the cavity of the brain into the abdomen. Antenatal screening allows parents the option of terminating the pregnancy. Research has revealed a link between folic-acid deficiency and spina bifida, and it is now common practice to prescribe this nutrient to expectant mothers. ●

I fell off our roof onto a flowerpot and fractured two vertebrae in my lower back, but I'm on my feet again only weeks later. Why wasn't I paralysed?

It sounds as though you cracked or chipped two vertebrae on the flowerpot. You were not paralysed because you did not damage your spinal cord. Fractures of the vertebrae more often result from a force acting up or down the spine which would increase the natural flexion of the spine, causing a 'burst' fracture.

A wedge-compression fracture may cause little disability and need no treatment, other than bed rest and physiotherapy, to strengthen and mobilize the back muscles and restore normal function. In burst fractures, however, one of the vertebral end-plates ruptures, forcing the intervertebral disk into the body of the vertebra. This creates a comminuted fracture (see Q 5), the fragments of which have burst out in all directions. A CT scan is performed to discover whether the spinal cord has been damaged by bits of the vertebral body being driven into it. If cord and nerves have escaped unscathed, the surgeon may stabilize the affected vertebrae or remove fragments in case they cause injury later.

Dislocation results from a more violent force which dislocates an intervertebral joint so that the body of one vertebra is pushed forwards onto the one below, usually damaging the spinal cord. Where the patient is not paralysed, he would undergo surgery to reduce and fix the disjointed parts. ●

**My wife tripped
while hanging out the
washing and cracked
three ribs, but our
doctor said there
was no treatment.
Is she right?**

I wonder which ribs your wife cracked? She could pinpoint the area of injury, which is painful to the touch and hurts when taking deep breaths. When your doctor examined her, she may have compressed her chest wall between her hands. This is a reliable test for fractured ribs, but x-rays should always be taken to confirm the diagnosis.

Most rib fractures heal spontaneously and serious displacement is rare, because the fragments are secured by intercostal muscles. The danger of displacement is that a fragment punctures a lung.

Treatment is needed to lessen the patient's pain and reduce the risk of complications. Most doctors prescribe simple anti-inflammatory medication and advise patients to do deep-breathing exercises for the first three weeks. This ensures that the lung area is fully expanded; important as shallow breathing increases the risk of infection.

Possible lung complications of fractured ribs, however, which includes bleeding into the chest or lung cavity, and possibly a collapsed lung are serious, and may prove fatal if prompt treatment is unavailable. Pneumonia is a possibility, especially in bed-ridden patients. All these occur most commonly after violent injuries to the chest wall, especially multiple rib fracture after, for instance, a road accident or other major incident.

47 My mother's father had 'bamboo spine'. What is this, and does it run in families?

Your grandfather had ankylosing spondylitis, a chronic inflammatory disease of the vertebrae and spinal ligaments that typically affects young men. Starting in the sacro-iliac joints (where the end of the spine articulates with the sides of the bony hipbone), the disease creeps up the spine to involve the lower and upper back and often the neck, with bony-bridged fixation of the joints.

The first signs are morning stiffness and a progressive loss of spinal movement. The disease tends to remain active for 10–15 years and then become quiescent. The cause is unknown, although it may be inherited and there is an established link with sero-negative chronic juvenile arthritis (*see Q 77*) in family members. Early symptoms include lower back pain and stiffness. There may be general pain down one or both legs, and all movements are limited in the affected area of the spine ('poker back'). Involvement of the upper spine results in greatly reduced chest expansion and sometimes chest pain.

There is no specific treatment, but non-steroidal anti-inflammatory drugs (NSAIDs) help to control the pain and stiffness. Special exercises help make the most of remaining movement, and patients are advised to sleep flat on their backs with a single pillow. An operation (wedge osteotomy) can correct this deformity where necessary. ●

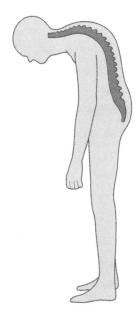

Ankylosing spondylitis is caused by the hardening of the cartilages in the spine. The bones slowly fuse together leading to the stooped posture and pain.

48 I'm 12 and may have
to have an operation
for curvature of the
spine in a year or so.
Will it hurt, and is it
really necessary?

It sounds as though you may have idiopathic structural scoliosis (*see Q 13*). Of its several forms, yours is the most important because, after starting in childhood or adolescence, it continues until growth stops in the mid or late teens. It could affect your growth and health later on, especially when it occurs in the upper back, unless it is treated.

When an operation is planned, this is usually because the outlook would otherwise be poor. Upper-back scoliosis – especially when it starts early – tends to worsen. The abnormal portion of the spine curves one way (the primary curve) and the adjoining area curves the other way to compensate.

Exercises have no effect on the underlying structural defect, but are useful for strengthening and toning the muscles. Surgery is usually postponed until the mid-teen years to minimize the loss of height that can result. Meanwhile an orthotic brace is usually prescribed and worn almost continuously.

The aim of the operation is to fuse the joints of all the vertebrae in the primary curve, after correcting the curvature as much as possible. This used to be achieved by traction (weights) or a plaster cast, but is now often carried out at the time of the operation. This may sound scary, but it is of course done under a general anaesthetic. You will have to wear a plaster jacket afterwards while the bones fuse together. ●

49 My nephew, who is 14, is very round-shouldered and often complains of backache. My sister took him to a specialist, who prescribed six weeks' bed-rest on a mattress on the floor. Is this really all he needs?

Your nephew has the symptoms of adolescent kyphosis (rounded upper back), an uncommon disorder affecting youngsters aged 13–16, who develop round shoulders and pain in the upper spine, with affected vertebrae feeling tender to the touch.

This disorder, also known as Scheuermann's disease, seems to spring from a fault in the ossification of the upper spine. Each vertebra ossifies (replaces cartilage with bone) at three points: a primary in the centre, and two secondaries that appear around puberty – one at the upper and lower end of each vertebra. These secondary centres become disturbed, with the result that the intervertebral discs become narrowed in front and the vertebral bodies slightly wedge-shaped.

Scheuermann's kyphosis remains active for one or two years, but the pain generally subsides after a few months, leaving varying degrees of rounded shoulders. The sole long-term complication is an increased risk of osteoarthritis in the affected joints later on. The only disease it may resemble is TB spine (tuberculous spondylitis), although blood tests and x-rays are good indicators of the differences.

Mild forms of the disease need no treatment, but rest on a flat, firm bed is usually recommended. A brace and physiotherapy may be prescribed, as well as exercise to strengthen the spinal muscles. ●

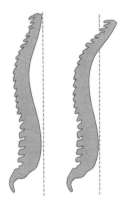

ABOVE LEFT *The normal curvature of the spine.* ABOVE RIGHT *The effects of kyphosis where the outward curve is exaggerated and the neck becomes convex.*

SCHEUERMANN'S DISEASE

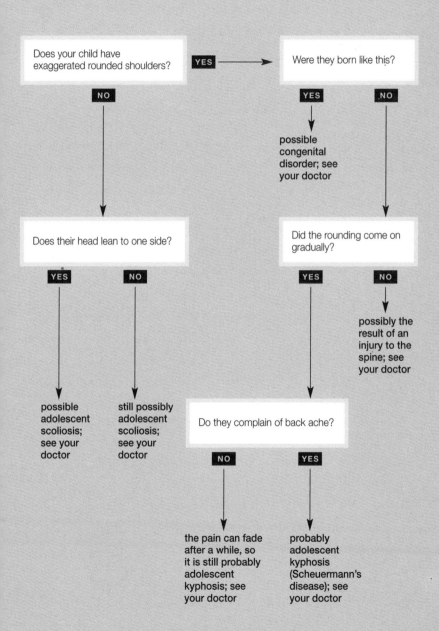

Does your child have exaggerated rounded shoulders?

YES → Were they born like this?

NO ↓

YES ↓
possible congenital disorder; see your doctor

NO ↓
Did the rounding come on gradually?

Does their head lean to one side?

YES ↓
possible adolescent scoliosis; see your doctor

NO ↓
still possibly adolescent scoliosis; see your doctor

YES ↓
Do they complain of back ache?

NO ↓
possibly the result of an injury to the spine; see your doctor

NO ↓
the pain can fade after a while, so it is still probably adolescent kyphosis; see your doctor

YES ↓
probably adolescent kyphosis (Scheuermann's disease); see your doctor

50 I suffered a slipped disk while moving some heavy furniture and was off work for a month. What exactly is this condition?

This is a prolapse (a bulging outwards) of the jelly-like filling within an intervertebral disk through a tear in the disk's tough fibrous casing (*see Q 37*). When it occurs in the lower back, the discs most likely to be affected are those between the fourth and fifth lumbar, or the fifth lumbar and first sacral, vertebrae. The disk-filling either stretches the major pain-sensitive ligament down the back of the spine, causing pain in the immediate area, or pushes right through it, pressing on nearby spinal nerves.

A prolapsed lumbar disk typically occurs between the ages of 18 and 60. While generally triggered by an injury or mechanical strain, degeneration is a risk factor among sufferers at the upper end of this age range. The pain, which can be agonizing, often starts suddenly a few hours or days after the incident, while the person is coughing, twisting round or stooping. At first unaided movement is impossible, but the acute pain subsides after a few days. It is then felt extending (as sciatica) in one or other buttock and down the back or side of the thigh to the calf or foot, and is aggravated by sudden jerking movements, such as those caused by coughing.

In the vast majority of cases bed-rest, possibly a surgical support corset and gentle exercise are the only treatment required. Healing occurs as the disk-filling shrinks and is converted to fibrous tissue.

51 I was bending down and suddenly got stuck – I just couldn't get up again until someone helped me, and I nearly vomited with the pain. What do you think caused this, and will it return?

Your symptoms sound like those of a prolapsed lumbar disk (*see Q 50*), but in your letter you say that no evidence of this condition was found. Acute lumbago is the name both doctors and patients use for lower back pain of the type you describe. It may be due to a number of causes.

It is possible that you sustained a relatively minor injury some time ago that ejected the jelly-like interior of a disk out of its normal position, but not far back enough to press upon a root of the sciatic nerve. In this situation sciatica would develop later.

Another possible explanation is a sudden nipping of the synovial membrane lining of one of the facet joints where two bony prominences of adjoining vertebrae fit together. Because synovial membrane is extremely pain-sensitive, this would cause heat, swelling and discomfort in the area, resulting in the type of pain you describe. Or it could be caused by a partial dislocation of a lumbar vertebra, with subsequent strain of the major pain-sensitive ligament going down the back of the spine.

The usual treatment is to rest the spine – either by bed-rest or by a plaster jacket or surgical corset, for 6–12 weeks, depending on progress. The sufferer usually recovers completely within one to two weeks, but many are so frightened by the severity of the pain that they need frequent reassessment. ●

Q

52

I am a 55-year-old shop assistant, and for the past six months I have been suffering from terrible pains in my right buttock after standing for an hour. I also notice this when I walk my dog. What is happening to me?

You sound as though you may have spinal stenosis syndrome (meaning narrowing of the spine), whereby standing and walking beyond a certain limit bring on increasingly severe pain in the buttocks and lower limbs on one or both sides of the body. Typically a heavy, aching sensation starts and grows until the person is obliged to sit down.

Most sufferers experience the problem after standing for a while. Relief comes only by sitting down or lying with the hips and knees drawn up in a sitting position. After a few minutes, the pain subsides enough for you to stand or walk again for a bit.

The dimensions of the spinal canal harbouring the spinal cord comprise the underlying problem in spinal stenosis. In the lumbar region these vary greatly between individuals, as does the cross-sectional shape of the canal, which is rounded in some people and triangular in others. Some people therefore have little room for manoeuvre at the lower part of their spinal canal, where the cord comes to an end as nerve strands called the *cauda equina* or 'horse's tail' (which it resembles).

Mild symptoms can be controlled by avoiding prolonged standing and by modifying your activities, (cycling instead of walking, for example). People with severe spinal stenosis may need an operation to decompress the segments of the spinal cord.

53 I am due to have a CT scan on my lower back. Is this a safe procedure?

CT stands for computerized tomography, a means of obtaining pictures of cross-sections of the body that are inaccessible to plain X-ray film. A computer then reconstructs series 'slices' (cross-sectons of your lower back) – 'cut', as it were, at varying depths from the surface – which appear on a specialized TV screen. These images result from the varying tissue densities within the area under investigation, being especially well marked where these densities vary most (for instance, bone and muscle). They also show changes in tissue density within a particular kind of tissue, indicating any disease process present.

You do not say why you are having your CT scan, but the spinal column and canal, the hipbone and its contents are often investigated by this method, especially when fractures or fracture-dislocations are present. This is a medical emergency and obviously does not apply in your case, but prompt information about the extent of the injury is vital in order to minimize damage to the central nervous system and the spinal nerves.

CT scans carry the same risks as X-rays (minimal in the hands of an experienced operator using properly maintained equipment and the standard safety precautions). Be sure to tell the radiographer or doctor if you suspect that you may be pregnant. ●

54 I have had an ache in my lower back since having my last child 15 years ago. Now it's with me almost all the time, especially after making beds, but my doctor says that there is nothing wrong. What do you think it could be?

Assuming that your doctor has carried out x-rays, blood tests and a pelvic scan to eliminate serious problems, you are probably suffering from postural backache (or chronic lower lumbar ligamentous strain). This is most common in women, who can often relate its onset to childbirth, an operation or a debilitating illness, although it may start for no apparent reason.

The pain – typically felt in the lower back – is aggravated by bending and stooping, and the diagnosis is made by default, since neither physical examination nor x-rays reveal any abnormality. You are more at risk if you are overweight, have flabby muscles due to lack of toning exercises or a debilitating illness, or have given birth to several children.

Nagging lower back pain may continue for many years despite treatment. Losing excess weight is often helpful, especially when combined with active exercises devised by a physiotherapist to strengthen the muscles of the spine. Heat and massage may be included in this treatment. Manipulation of the spine and sacro-iliac joints (*see page 140*) can help patients who are neither elderly nor frail. If none of these measures brings relief, your doctor may prescribe a reinforced corset. The support it offers can make life bearable, especially if you are overweight and have gained no relief from physiotherapy. ●

I sat down hard on a concrete floor, bruising my tailbone. It's now torture to sit down, and even opening my bowels is painful. Should I have an x-ray?

You should if the pain continues for weeks or months without improving. If the x-ray results are negative and no underlying abnormality can be found, you would then have coccydynia (a painful coccyx or tailbone) diagnosed. In severe cases it is normal for the area to be tender to the touch and for the pain to be increased by sitting down or passing motions, but relieved by standing or lying down. The discomfort may extend upwards between the buttocks into the mid-region of the lower part of the spine, as well as into the back wall of the hipbone rim.

Bruising of the membrane covering the sacrum or coccyx, or a strain of the sacro-coccygygial joint, is usually responsible, but a doctor will want to exclude other causes. Besides x-rays, this would require an internal examination of the back passage, an attempt to move the coccyx gently to see if this reproduced the pain and/or a CT scan.

The symptoms eventually subside of their own accord. Manipulation, short-wave electrical-current therapy and hydrocortisone injections work for some people, but not others; in exceptionally persistent cases the coccyx can be surgically removed. Many sufferers gain relief from using a cushion to lessen the discomfort of sitting, and twice-daily applications of herbal comfrey ointment (avoiding any lacerations, and the skin on and around the anus). ●

Upper limbs

Injuries to the upper limbs range from a dislocated shoulder to fractures of the collar bone, the point of the elbow or the wrist. Together with these injuries this section also discusses ailments such as 'tennis elbow', 'frozen shoulder' and 'trigger finger', and looks at what the funny bone is, how the shoulder joint works and at various conditions that may affect the hands.

56 I am 47 and my shoulder has hurt for the past six months, but x-rays didn't reveal anything. What could this be?

Since you do not mention injury, the symptoms suggest 'frozen' shoulder, a condition that causes considerable pain and stiffness, but no recognizable changes on x-ray film. The cause is unknown, but neither infection nor trauma can be held responsible and the discomfort gradually disappears with effective treatment.

Frozen shoulder starts gradually, and for no apparent reason, with a severe ache in the upper arm. The actions that you will find most painful are those involving the head of your upper arm bone moving within the saucer-shaped glenoid cavity on the side of your shoulder girdle – actions that may be reduced to about one-quarter or half of their normal range. With your arm hanging down by your side as you stand upright, these include lifting your arm out sideways until level with your shoulder (abduction);

bringing your arm in an upwards direction, close to your body (flexion); raising your hand in the air as high as it will go (extension); and turning your arm and hand first inwards as far as possible, then outwards in the opposite direction, with a corkscrew-like motion (rotation).

The underlying problem is not yet understood, but is probably due to a loss of resilience or 'give' within the joint capsule (the outer fibrous envelope encasing the joint), complicated by adhesions formed between the folds of synovial membrane in the shoulder joint's interior. Suitable treatment in the early, most painful stages consists of rest in a sling, which is removed for short periods every day to allow gentle exercises to be practised. Simple analgesics and non-steroidal anti-inflammatory drugs (NSAIDs) can provide much relief. As the pain lessens you will be encouraged to increase the exercises until you have regained full shoulder-joint movement. Gentle manipulation by a physiotherapist during the early stages can help. ●

My father, aged 65, slipped while climbing a tree and strained his shoulder. Now he has difficulty raising his arm. Can anything be done?

It sounds as though your father has torn his shoulder tendons. The tendons of the muscles around the upper back and shoulder blade unite to make a cuff over the shoulder, blending with the joint's capsule. Under a sudden, violent strain (which generally results from a fall) this cuff gives way, tearing close to the capsule that it usually involves. The edges of the rent pull apart, leaving a gaping hole forming a tunnel between the interior of the shoulder joint and a little pocket underlying the shoulder-joint tip of the shoulder blade.

This injury happens most often in someone aged 60 or over. The most common symptoms are pain at the tip of the shoulder and down the arm, and difficulty in arm-raising. The most tender point is high up on the shoulder below the margins of the acromion (part of the shoulder blade). When the patient attempts to lift his arm above his head, no movement occurs in the usual region between the head of the long arm bone and its shallow socket, on the side of the pectoral girdle.

Instead, movement of the shoulder blade can lift the arm 45–60 degrees away from the side of the body and, if the patient allows someone to hold his arm and lift it passively more than 90 degrees away from the side of his body, he can raise it the rest of the way into a fully upright position by the action of his deltoid muscles, which are situated just below the shoulder joint in his upper arm.

Doctors diagnose torn shoulder tendons from the characteristic movements of the joint and, where the tear is complete, from the communicating channel between the joint's interior and the sac shown on an ultrasound scan or an arthrogram (a picture of the joint's inside obtained by special x-ray). Surgical repair of the torn tendon is more successful in young patients with healthy, strong tendons, who can passively move their shoulder during the first few days, but they must avoid active attempts to raise their arm for a month. Older people usually find that their disability lessens with time. Sometimes the action of their deltoid muscles alone comes to restore normal function. ●

58 I couldn't take my eyes off the massive shoulders of the shot-putters in the Sydney Olympics. How is the shoulder joint constructed?

The shoulder joint is one of the most versatile in the human body, and the most unstable. It dislocates more often than all the other joints put together. It is a synovial ball-and-socket joint (see page 80) formed by the head of the upper arm bone articulating with the shallow, saucer-shaped glenoid cavity on the side of the shoulder blade. Its capsule is reinforced from above and the sides by fibrous slips from nearby muscles, but it is thin and lax in comparison with that of the hip, thereby allowing the shoulder joint its wide range of movement.

The capsule has little support from below, and is placed under great strain when the arm is raised sideways at right-angles to the body, but is further strengthened by ligaments. The three weak bands of the glenohumeral ligament run from the lip of the glenoid cavity to various positions on the upper end of the upper arm bone. The more important (because more powerful) coracohumeral ligament helps to limit movements that rotate the arm outwards from the shoulder in an anticlockwise direction, as well as movements bringing the arm close in to the side of the body.

The muscles of the upper arm and pectoral girdle, which are hugely developed in shot-putters and similar athletes, give the shoulder what little stability it possesses. Four short muscles inserted around the head of the upper arm bone are most important in 'holding the joint together'. In wide movements of the shoulder, especially, these work in unison to keep the head of the upper arm bone in position in the glenoid cavity, while the larger muscles surrounding the joint perform the movements, and prevent the capsule from dipping down onto the articulating surfaces, where it would get caught or come out of the socket and be badly dislocated. ●

Each throw of a shot-putter is dependent upon the interplay of bones, muscles and ligaments in the shoulder.

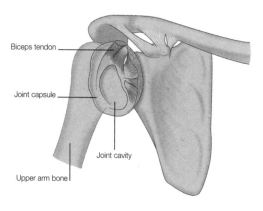

Biceps tendon

Joint capsule

Joint cavity

Upper arm bone

Q

59 I'm 13, and I broke my collar bone ice-skating. My mother made a fuss when the casualty officer just put my arm in a sling. Was this the right treatment?

An arm sling is the usual treatment for a fractured collar bone. This is why. You can feel – and see – your collar bone at the top of your chest, just below the hollow to the side of your neck. This slightly curved 'long' bone (*see below*) articulates with the upper end of your breastbone at one end, and with part of the shoulder blade at the other.

A direct blow onto the point of the shoulder causes 90 per cent of fractures to the collar bone. Falling onto an outstretched hand, transmitting force up the arm, accounts for nearly all the rest. The break usually happens in the outer third of the bone near the shoulder joint, and greenstick injuries are common (*see Q 4*). Often a slightly irregularity in the collar bone's outline is the only sign of damage – plus pain and swelling in the affected area.

The object of treatment is to make the patient more comfortable by taking the weight off the shoulder joint, where an important attachment has been lost. A wide arm sling, worn for a week or two, achieves this best. The old treatment of holding the shoulders braced back by a figure-of-eight bandage is rarely used these days, because of possible interference with the veins returning blood from the upper limb, or damage to one or more of the nerve trunks in the armpit. The broken bone ends usually remain sufficiently in place for healing to occur.

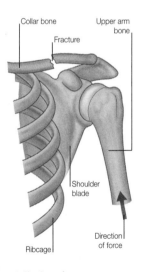

Collar bone fractures are very common, particularly among children. Most fractures here are due to extreme weight and pressure being put on the arm during a fall.

60 My doctor told me I had tennis elbow, but how could I have? I don't play tennis.

Tennis elbow (known medically as extensor tendinitis) is a common condition causing pain on the outer side of the elbow and often down the back of the forearm. It is probably due to strain of the extensor muscles in the forearm, followed by the repair of disrupted small blood vessels (capillaries, arterioles and venules) supplying the injured area. It can follow tennis or similar racket games, but in your case some other activity must be to blame. Unaccustomed exercise, such as carpentry or house-painting, is a common cause.

The defect lies outside the elbow joint, which retains its full range of movement and is unaffected. You can easily locate the problem area just in front of the outer epicondyle of the upper arm bone – this can be felt, and usually seen, as a bony knobble below the skin, x-rays look normal and there is no evidence of any disease process. A partial rupture doubtless occurs in the connective tissue fibres where the extensor muscles originate, an area that is rich in pain-sensitive nerve endings.

As you may have discovered, the discomfort is aggravated by putting these muscles on the stretch – that is, by lifting the arm with the palm of the hand facing downwards, a movement which normally occurs when pouring out tea, turning a stiff door handle or shaking hands.

Humerus

Area of tenderness

Tennis elbow may have very little to do with tennis but is due to a problem with the tendons of the elbow.

Left alone, tennis elbow almost invariably clears up, but it can persist for more than two years. Rest, or avoiding the activity for a while, allows the tissue to heal. Patients in need of treatment are usually prescribed a course of non-steroidal anti-inflammatory drugs (NSAIDs, *see Q 84*), but an injection of hydrocortisone, combined with local anaesthetic, into the tenderest spot is more effective. This is not an easy procedure, because the injection has to hit the spot precisely, and two or more shots are occasionally needed, at fortnightly intervals, before success is achieved. The area often feels worse for about 24 hours before the pain gradually diminishes, then disappears altogether. Surgery (carried out in only the most severe cases) consists of detaching the extensor fibres from their origin.

61 My mother's large dog pulled her over, and she's broken the point of her elbow. She's in her seventies. Will it heal?

This is a nasty fracture, especially in an older person, since it almost invariably results from a fall, causing the sufferer both upset and shock, and the pain can be severe.

Two types of fracture may be found in this area: a comminuted fracture (*see Q 5*), which is due to a direct blow or fall onto the elbow; and a clean transverse (straight-across) break, known as a traction lesion, when the patient falls onto the hand while the triceps muscle (at the back of the upper arm) is contracted, causing a break.

One clue as to which fracture your mother suffered is whether or not she is able to straighten her arm against resistance (an examining technique). If she can, then her fracture was comminuted – a diagnosis also suggested by bruising or grazing over the site of the injury. If she cannot, then she will have had a transverse fracture; you may also be able to feel a gap where the break occurred, when the swelling has gone down.

Comminuted fractures are treated by means of rest until the acute pain has subsided, then active movement is encouraged, possibly with the aid of a physiotherapist. Transverse fractures in which the bone fragments are not at all displaced are immobilized by being placed in a plaster cast for two to three weeks, after which exercises are begun. If the fragments are displaced, however, it becomes necessary to repair the triceps mechanism, realigning the bones and holding them in position by means of either surgical screws or wire.

A comminuted fracture of the elbow is treated by rest until the pain subsides following which specially designed exercises help strengthen the bone.

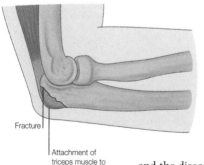

Fracture

Attachment of triceps muscle to olecranon process

There is no reason why your mother's fracture should not heal with satisfactory treatment, provided her bones are not too affected by osteoporosis, although non-union is a recognized complication of this injury. She may already have osteoarthritis in some of her joints, and the disease then predictably spreads to joints where serious damage has occurred. ●

The specialist diagnosed my sore shoulder as painful arc syndrome. He tried to explain this to me, but I didn't understand it.

Descriptions of this condition vary from simple to complex. Essentially you are experiencing pain in the shoulder and over the deltoid muscle that caps the top of the arm. It tends to be worse at night (varying from mild to excruciating), and is aggravated by actions such as putting on a jacket. Your shoulder looks normal, but there is a tender spot just below the acromion (part of the shoulder blade). On raising your arm sideways, the pain worsens between 45 and 120 degrees (the painful arc). Repeating the movement with your arm fully rotated outwards (anti-clockwise) may be far less painful to you.

If you have had this condition for long, you may have some muscle wasting and weakness, and raising your arm at the side, and rotating it outwards as described above, may be especially difficult.

Even in a normal shoulder, the clearance between the top end of the upper arm bone and the acromion is small when the arm is elevated sideways between 45 and 160 degrees. So any swollen, tender structure underneath the acromion is likely to be painfully pinched during this movement range, but return to relative normality when the arm is in the neutral position (hanging down by the side) or fully raised. This is the basis of painful arc syndrome, and five defects can give rise to it.

Three involve the supraspinatus muscle, which passes from the upper part of the shoulder blade over the shoulder into the greater tuberosity (roughened area) on the top part of the upper arm bone. A minor tear or strain, degeneration or a calcified deposit in its tendon can all cause tenderness and swelling. Fourthly, the small fibrous sac under the acromion can become inflamed by mechanical stress; and lastly, bruising or an undisplaced fracture of the greater tuberosity of the shoulder blade may be to blame. Treatment consists of rest in a sling, and specific exercises. Surgery to remove part of the acromion and eliminate pinching may be necessary to relieve severe long-term pain.

Q

63 **What exactly is the funny-bone in the elbow? How does this joint work?**

The so-called 'funny-bone' is actually the ulnar nerve which, on its way down the arm from the upper spine to the hand, appears behind the inner epicondyle of the upper arm bone. Covered only by skin, it can easily be rolled under the finger against the underlying bone. A blow or knock causes the characteristically sharp, tingling sensation we associate with this area.

The elbow joint itself consists of the lower rounded part and the irregular prominence of the upper arm bone articulating with the groove of the ulna and the head of the radius (the two bones of the forearm). It is a hinge joint surrounded by a capsule that is strengthened by two ligaments. The elbow is capable of two movements, flexion (drawing the forearm up towards the shoulder) and extension (straightening the elbow). The flexor muscles, including the biceps, are nearly twice as powerful as the extensors, and this is why, following a stroke, the forearm becomes flexed.

When the elbow is fully flexed, further movement is prevented by the forearm pressing upon the upper arm and by tension of the muscles and ligaments on the back of the joint. In full extension, the olecranon process of the ulna fits into a groove of the same name on the back of the upper arm bone, mechanically preventing any further movement, although this is not normally put to the test because of the tension within the capsule on the elbow's front.

The shape of the irregular prominence of the upper arm bone has the effect of pushing the ulna, and with it the forearm, slightly sideways when the arm is fully extended. Thus the upper arm and forearm are not in the same straight line, but form an angle – more prominent in women than in men – called the 'carrying angle', which disappears when the forearm is fully flexed. ●

I've just broken my wrist, and the doctor called it a Colles fracture. Is this serious?

Your injury is actually just above your wrist, being a break straight across the lower end of your radius. Sometimes this is a simple crack with no displacement of the fragments; but in the great majority of cases there is a characteristic deformity, due to the lower end of the radius being displaced in such a way that its articular surface faces downwards and backwards, instead of downwards and slightly forwards. It is also driven upwards and impacted into the upper fragment. A small peak of bone at the lower end of the ulna is often detached as well.

The altered contour is called a 'dinner fork' deformity, as this is what it resembles. Colles fractures are seen more often than any other injury in fracture clinics. They are uncommon in young adults, but by far the most common fractures in people over 40, especially in women, who run a higher risk of osteoporosis from the menopause onwards. Most Colles fractures result from a fall onto an outstretched hand.

Undisplaced (or only very slightly displaced) fractures are splinted in a plaster slab wrapped around the upper surface of the wrist and forearm, then bandaged firmly in position. Displaced fractures have to be reduced under anaesthesia; the hand is grasped firmly and traction is applied along the length of the bone to disimpact the fracture. The

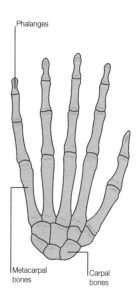

Phalanges

Metacarpal bones

Carpal bones

The hand derives stability from closely grouped carpal bones at the wrist joint, and flexibility from the metacarpals and phalanges whose joints permit a wide range of movement.

broken-off lower end of the radius is then pushed into place by pressing firmly on the back of the wrist with the thumbs while holding the front of the forearm with the fingers. After the position is checked by x-ray, a plaster slab is then applied from just below the elbow to the palm of the hand, with the wrist in a neutral or slightly flexed position.

You must attend for a further x-ray position check ten days after the above procedure, because the fracture can redisplace and may need repositioning. You can expect to wear your plaster for six weeks, and you will be encouraged to exercise your fingers, elbow and shoulder muscles. The chief complications include failure to unite (many patients accept a slight deformity in preference to undergoing further manipulation), and rupture of the long extensor tendon of the thumb a few weeks after the accident. The frayed tendon is difficult to suture, and a tendon transplant may be required.

65 A large round swelling has come up on the back of my husband's wrist, but I can't persuade him to go to our doctor. What could it be?

It sounds as if your husband has a ganglion (plural: ganglia), a cystic swelling at the back of the wrist that affects adults of all ages. Ganglia crop up less commonly at the front of the wrist, and occasionally in the palm and fingers. They rarely cause symptoms (although large ones can be mildly uncomfortable) and are harmless, with no links to cancer. Some feel soft to the touch, but more often they are tense and firm. The hard ones may be mistaken for a bony tumour, but a doctor examining the growth carefully will always pick up the slight 'give' of the ganglion's walls due to the fluid interior.

Opinion is divided about the causes. Some experts believe ganglia to be simply a sign of degeneration, while others are convinced that they are benign tumours of a tendon sheath or joint capsule. They have a wall of fibrous tissue, and while they are connected at some point with a joint's capsule or a tendon sheath, no communication channel exists between the cyst and these structures. They contain clear viscous fluid, which sometimes allows the ganglion to be dispersed by firm pressure. This manoeuvre, while not in itself painful, is of limited use because the ganglion often slowly reforms.

The only complication is mechanical pressure on surrounding structures from ganglia that are deeply situated in the wrist or palm. The median and ulnar nerves and their branches then show signs of disturbed function – that is, loss of sensation and weakened muscular movement.

Some doctors prefer to treat ganglia by aspiration – drawing off their fluid content with a wide-bore needle. The question of surgical excision can be deferred for the few ganglia that appear in children, because they often disappear spontaneously, but should be performed without delay when symptoms of nerve pressure exist. ●

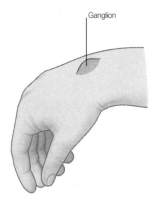

Ganglion

A ganglion is a smooth-walled cyst arising from the tendons supplying the fingers and hand. It may cause pressure discomfort, but is entirely harmless and not cancerous.

My father-in-law, aged 60, has had a lump on his right palm for some months and now he's having difficulty straightening his fingers. He claims it doesn't hurt, but my mother-in-law is worried sick. What is this?

He has a condition named Dupuytren's (pronounced doo-pee-trons) contracture, which starts in the sheet of connective tissue in the palm of the hand. This is normally a tough, thin membrane immediately below the skin, with fibres radiating from the front of the wrist to insertions into the first and second small bones of the fingers. When Dupuytren's develops, this tissue becomes greatly thickened and gradually contracts, drawing down and flexing the fingers at their first and second joints (the knuckle joints, and the set beyond these).

The tissue below the fourth and fifth fingers is most affected, and it is these fingers that undergo the worst flexion-deformity. The joints are untouched at first, but eventually develop contractures as their capsules thicken and change. This disorder can attack the tissue on the sole of the foot, and the penis. Widespread contractural deformities are known as Dupuytren's disease.

Its cause is unknown, although it is much more common in men and tends to run in families. Injury may act as a trigger, and epileptics are more at risk. The only effective treatment is surgical excision of the thickened part of the tissue, but this is not necessary for slight disease, especially in an elderly person.

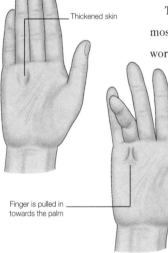

Thickened skin

Finger is pulled in towards the palm

In the early stages of Dupuytren's contracture the skin of the palm becomes thickened. This increases until the fingers are drawn towards the palm of the hand.

Q

My father tripped three months ago and broke his scaphoid bone. It hasn't mended, and now he will have to have an operation. Wasn't it set correctly?

Your father was unfortunate – the scaphoid (meaning boat-shaped) bone generally heals readily enough, but there is a greater risk of non-union than in most other bones. A fractured scaphoid (one of the eight wrist bones) is common in young adults, but far less common in children and elderly people. The usual cause is a fall onto an outstretched hand, breaking the bone straight across the middle, leaving fragments of approximately equal size, usually without displacement. The fracture is often overlooked, either because the wrist was not x-rayed or the fracture was missed. The discomfort is usually slight and the patient may fail to seek medical attention because he mistakes his injury for a sprain.

Suspicious signs include imperfect wrist movements and tenderness on pressure over the anatomical snuffbox (a small depression at the base of the thumb). Uncomplicated scaphoid fractures are treated by immobilizing the wrist in plaster until x-rays confirm union, usually within two to three months. Delayed union is treated surgically by screwing the fragments together, then grafting in small bone slivers to fill any gaps. Tissue death, due to inadequate blood supply, may happen when the blood vessels to a fragment are damaged by a break. The only treatment is removal of the dead bone and, sometimes, replacement with a prosthesis. ●

My uncle says that only people who use guns get 'trigger fingers', but I'm sure he's off the mark! Who is right?

You are. The cause of trigger finger, a disorder of the flexor tendons of the finger joints, is unknown, although the mechanism seems clear. The first part of the fibrous sheath around the flexor tendons at the base of a finger or thumb becomes thickened, narrowing the mouth of the sheath. The tendons within become 'waisted' opposite the constriction, and swollen just before it. The swollen segment then has difficulty entering the mouth of the sheath when the person attempts to straighten his or her fingers from the flexed position.

This is a fairly common condition in the fingers of middle-aged people (women especially) and in the thumbs of babies and small children. Adults complain of soreness at the base of affected fingers, and of the fingers locking when flexed. Often a small tender swelling can be felt at the base of the finger.

Infants and children with this condition are unable to straighten their thumb, which remains locked in flexion. It is often impossible to straighten the thumb manually, even using moderate force. As with the adult form, a small swelling may be located at the base of the digit, although the characteristic snapping sound is rarely present. Both the infantile and adult forms can be corrected by a simple operation in which the mouth of the fibrous flexor sheaths are cut open lengthways. ●

Lower limbs

Fractures and sprains of the lower limbs and joints – the legs, hips, knees and ankles – are common among the elderly and those who exercise aggressively. The feet may also give rise to a number of different complaints, ranging from ingrowing toenails and bunions to stress fractures and inflammation of the sole of the foot. This section looks in detail at many of these conditions.

69 My granny, a fit 72, died after breaking her hip. Why did this happen?

Broken hips claim many lives, not least because they usually occur in frail, elderly people (*see* Qs 16 and 26), often living alone. Typically the person (most often a woman) trips and falls and cannot get up unaided. When helped to her feet, she cannot put any weight on the affected leg, which tends to turn outwards at an abnormal angle. The shock of falling, compounded by the pain, possible hypothermia or dehydration if not found for hours, removal to hospital and surgery can all have adverse effects. Complications of the fracture and extended bed-rest pose further risks.

Generally the long thigh bone, when weakened by osteoporosis, breaks at its neck – the angled portion bearing the rounded head that articulates with the saucer-shaped cavity on the side of the hipbone. Fat globules from the bone marrow can escape into the bloodstream and reach the pulmonary circulation, blocking blood flow to the lungs. This condition – called pulmonary embolism – can also arise from a fragment of blood clot reaching the lungs from a deep-vein thrombosis (DVT) in the lower limbs. This is a potential risk for anyone confined to bed for a significant period, especially an elderly person who may already suffer from poor circulation. Bed-rest also weakens the bones and leg muscles, increasing the likelihood of further stumbles and falls and, therefore, further fractures.

Finally, repair is itself traumatic. General anaesthesia carries its own risks; some surgeons reunite the head and neck by fixing them internally with a compression screw-plate or a nail and plate, after flexing and rotating the thigh to reduce the fracture (that is, correctly reposition the broken fragments). In patients over the age of 70, however, it is common to excise the broken part and replace it with a metal prosthesis (replacement arthroplasty), sometimes inserting a plastic socket as well (total replacement arthroplasty), especially if the bones are very soft. Arthroplasties are somewhat severe on the patient, but the results are more satisfactory than those of internal fixation, especially in elderly patients who are unlikely to give their new hip joint too much hard wear. ●

Q

70 My sprained ankle has taken six weeks to heal. Is this unusual?

Two types of ankle injury are loosely termed a 'sprain', and you are pretty certain to have suffered the more serious of them. The focus of damage is the lateral ligament, which strengthens and protects the ankle's outer aspect. It runs down in three thick strands from the prominent bony knobble on the outer ankle, to join onto the ankle bone and the heel bones in the foot. One of these strands is the one usually torn in a sprained ankle.

Typically, the person stumbles, landing on a twisted foot turned inwards. The ankle swells rapidly around the calf bone's lower end, the pain is severe and walking difficult. In a simple sprain, the lateral ligament is partly torn, and slight bruising appears a day or two later. X-rays look normal, eliminating bony injury, and the examining doctor can turn the patient's foot slightly inwards. Simple sprains are treated with a crêpe support bandage for up to two weeks, and the patient advised to exercise freely.

A more violent injury may rupture the lateral ligament, tilting and partly dislocating the ankle bone within its joint. The pain and swelling are more severe, the bruising more intense, and the patient can rarely put his foot to the ground. Ligaments that fail to heal can lead to recurrent dislocation of the ankle bone, resulting in the ankle being put in a below-knee plaster for at least six weeks.

I am 56 and recently started doing some regular brisk walking. Now I have a very sore place on the top of my foot, and every movement hurts. Could this be cancer?

Your symptoms are not in the least suggestive of cancer, but do suggest a stress fracture, a common injury among athletes and people taking up unaccustomed brisk exercise. Your variety, fatigue fracture, often affects the long bones of the foot when repetitive stress is applied by walking and so on.

Known risk factors include increasing age, being a woman, being white, lack of fitness, and a menstrual history of low oestrogen production and late onset of periods at puberty. Muscle fatigue is a further trigger. Rigid, high foot arches absorb energy poorly, predisposing to stress fractures, while flat, flexible feet absorb energy well, reducing the risk.

Your pain is typical in following a major change in exercise routine and in worsening with continued use. An examination of your foot might reveal a spindle-shaped soft-tissue swelling over the fractured bone, although x-ray confirmation may be impossible. Although stress fractures can affect almost any bone, only around 33 per cent appear on x-ray in the early stages, and only about 67 per cent do so later on. A bone scan is the standard for stress-fracture diagnosis.

Like most stress fractures, yours should heal within six weeks if you keep generally active and avoid brisk walking until the pain ceases. Correct shoes and walking surface, and possibly orthotic foot supports, may help prevent a recurrence.

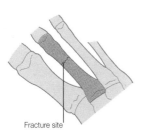

Fracture site

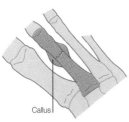

Callus

A stress fracture in the shaft of a long bone such as a metatarsal, may not appear in an x-ray until the protective layer (callus) is laid down to strengthen the cracked area.

STRESS FRACTURE

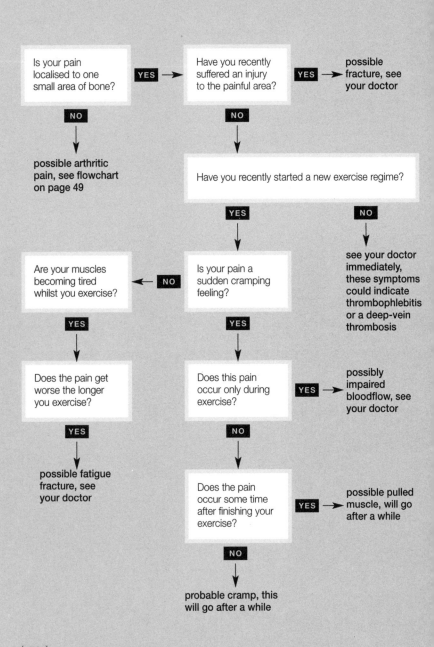

Is your pain localised to one small area of bone?

YES → Have you recently suffered an injury to the painful area?

YES → possible fracture, see your doctor

NO ↓

possible arthritic pain, see flowchart on page 49

NO ↓

Have you recently started a new exercise regime?

YES ↓

NO ↓

see your doctor immediately, these symptoms could indicate thrombophlebitis or a deep-vein thrombosis

Are your muscles becoming tired whilst you exercise?

← **NO** — Is your pain a sudden cramping feeling?

YES ↓

YES ↓

Does the pain get worse the longer you exercise?

Does this pain occur only during exercise?

YES → possibly impaired bloodflow, see your doctor

YES ↓

possible fatigue fracture, see your doctor

NO ↓

Does the pain occur some time after finishing your exercise?

YES → possible pulled muscle, will go after a while

NO ↓

probable cramp, this will go after a while

Our granddaughter, aged six, has been complaining of a pain in her right hip and groin, and recently started to limp. What could be causing this?

Your granddaughter's hip and groin pain, and her limp, are typical of Perthe's disease, an abnormality of bone development at the upper end of the head of the thighbone. Known medically as osteochondritis juvenilis, this disease can affect other parts of the skeleton, and involves a bony growth centre temporarily softening and becoming deformed by pressure. The disease lasts for about three years, by which time the bone has rehardened. Its cause is unknown, but a temporary interruption of the blood supply to the affected area is thought to be responsible for it.

Perthe's disease mainly affects children between the ages of five and ten. It has no direct effect on general health, the main risk being to the affected hip joint, since a permanently misshapen thighbone head increases the risk of osteoarthritis later on. If part of the head escapes deformity, the outlook is favourable, but if the whole of the upper end is affected, the thighbone head may enlarge and become seriously flattened. Meanwhile the saucer-shaped cavity on the side of the pelvis, with which the thighbone forms the hip joint, tends to follow the contours of the thighbone head as it grows, becoming abnormally large and shallow. The affected limb may become shorter than the unaffected one, although never seriously so.

The present trend is to regulate treatment according to likely outcome, judging from the shape of the thighbone head as it appears on x-rays in the early stages. Children in the 'favourable outcome' group do not usually require treatment apart from a few weeks' rest to allow the pain to subside, although it is vital that they have regular x-ray reviews; those in the 'unfavourable' group need treatment aimed at 'containment' of the thighbone head within the saucer-shaped cavity, which then acts as a mould for the softened bone. This can be achieved by splinting the limbs at appropriate angles, or by an operation to reposition the two components of the hip joint. ●

73 **My nephew, aged 14, has a sore knee and the doctor said it was Osgood-Schlatter's disease. Is this serious?**

This complaint was once thought to be a form of osteochondritis juvenilis (*see Q 72*), but experts now agree that Osgood-Schlatter's disease is no more than a strain of the shinbone tubercle, a bony prominence at the front upper end of the shinbone into which the kneecap tendon is inserted.

The disease affects children between 10 and 14, and is more common in boys. The pain is felt just below the kneecap, which is embedded in the lower part of the tendon of the muscle on the thigh front. Strenuous activity aggravates the soreness, as does tensing this muscle (which doctors test by asking the patient to lie on his back and raise his straightened leg against resistance from the examiner's hand).

The kneecap causes the muscle to pull on the shinbone at an angle, considerably increasing its power and thereby the forces at work on the unfused tubercle, which is tender to the touch. The knee joint itself is normal and x-rays show only an enlarged tubercle, sometimes broken into pieces. Few children need treatment for Osgood-Schlatter's disease, which invariably clears up, although this takes time and parents are often advised to restrict activities such as football and cycling. If (unusually) the pain is severe, the knee should be rested for two months in a plaster cylinder from groin to ankle. ●

74 My knees are swollen and painful after kneeling on church floors, taking brass rubbings. What has happened to them?

You have 'housemaid's knee', so called because it often afflicted housemaids who spent hours on their hands and knees scrubbing. The medical name is pre-patellar bursitis, caused by inflammation of a small fibrous sac in front of the kneecap.

Yours is the irritative kind, caused by repeated friction. The fibrous walls of the sac thicken, and the sac fills with fluid. The skin over your knee will be swollen and painful. If you prod it gently with your fingertips, you will feel its fluctuating interior. This is not a form of arthritis, and the knee joint itself is not involved. You will be able to take up your hobby again when the swelling has subsided, but avoid kneeling for the present and ensure that in future you have a soft cushion to kneel on.

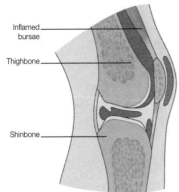

Inflamed bursae

Thighbone

Shinbone

Bursitis affects the small fluid filled sacks which normally reduce the friction in a joint. These become inflammed and swollen as the production of fluid increases.

Treatment includes a simple analgesic or anti-inflammatory. Doctors can draw the fluid off the front of the knee using a local anaesthetic, if the trouble persists. If it returns, the sac can be removed in a simple operation under general anaesthetic.

The other variety (suppurative pre-patellar bursitis) is caused by infection with pus-producing organisms, which reach the fibrous sac via a puncture wound on the front of the knee or an infected wound in the leg. The wall of the sac becomes acutely inflamed, the sac itself full of pus and the area most painful. This is treated with antibiotics and analgesics, and drained by incision.

Q

75 Two days after my baby was born the doctor laid her down and bent her hips forward, making her cry. He said he was 'listening for clicks'. Whatever did he mean?

The doctor was examining your baby for dislocated hips. Congenital (present at birth) hip dislocation or instability can nearly always be detected shortly after birth. This test, called the Barlow manoeuvre, is part of the repertoire to which most new babies are subject.

Facing the child's genitals, the doctor takes hold of the upper part of each thigh between fingers (behind) and thumb (in front), while the baby's hips are flexed at right-angles and the knees are fully bent. While each thigh in turn is firmly pressed downwards towards the couch, the middle finger presses forward behind a bony prominence on the upper end of the thighbone, and alternately the thumb in front presses backwards.

Most babies cry when this test is performed, but it is uncomfortable rather than painful and can pick up two important abnormalities. A dislocated thighbone head returns to the saucer-shaped cavity on the side of the hipbone with a palpable and audible 'click'; and the backwards pressure from the thumb temporarily dislocates an unstable joint. The results of other hip-movement tests are combined with those of the Barlow manoeuvre to obtain as clear a picture as possible of the hips' normality.

Congenital dislocation of the hips develops either in the uterus or during birth. It is one of the most common birth deformities, and early diagnosis is essential in order to avoid lifetime crippling. Girls are affected six times more often than boys, and one-third of babies who suffer from this abnormality have both hips affected. Unless it is detected in infancy it may pass unnoticed until the child starts to walk and as a result the child either waddles or limps.

The Barlow manoeuvre tests for hip abnormalities in the newly born. The doctor pushes the hips through their full range of movement listening for clicks which signal a congenital dislocation.

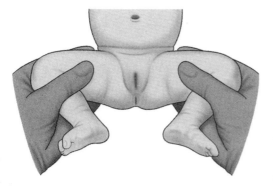

It is important that any congenital dislocations are found early so that the child can learn to walk without limping and their legs can grow straight.

Q

76 I do meals-on-wheels, and was shocked to notice that the large toenail of an elderly client had grown up like a sheep's horn, about7.5cm/3in high. Could this be cancerous?

No, what you observed was not cancer but a condition called onychogryposis, which (translated from the Greek) means 'hooked nail'. It usually affects the large toe, the nail of which becomes hugely overgrown, thickened and curved, like a sheep's horn. In itself it is harmless and painless, but of course it prevents the sufferer from wearing properly protective outdoor shoes; this, in turn, can lead to soft-tissue injury and other damage.

As a temporary measure, this condition can be treated by removing the nail under a local anaesthetic, but the new nail will develop just like the old one. The only permanent cure is surgical destruction of the nail bed.

Another condition, this time involving nail undergrowth, is a below-the-nail bony outgrowth. This develops on the upper surface of the last segment of a toe – again, usually the large toe. It projects forwards and upwards between the tip of the toenail and the soft tissue that this shelters. The nail is lifted up and becomes deformed, while the skin of the soft tissue overlying the outgrowth becomes coarse and hard. Pressing upon the nail or last segment of soft tissue causes sharp pain, and the outgrowth can clearly be seen on side-view x-rays of the foot. This condition is yet another impediment to the wearing of outdoor shoes.

Finally, toenails can ingrow. The nail burrows down into the nail groove, where pressure ulcerates the soft tissue, which then grows over the nail. Initial treatment teaches the patient to cut the toenails squarely, to insert some cotton wool under the ingrowing edges of the nails and to keep the feet extremely clean and dry. Secondly, a narrow wedge of soft tissue alongside the ingrowing nail is removed, and a segment of fine polythene tubing that has been cut in half lengthways is inserted there. Ultimately the matrix from which the toenails develop may have to be removed.

Q

77 **My right foot is very sore underneath the heel; I can hardly bear to put my foot to the ground. What do you think is wrong?**

This sounds like plantar (meaning sole of the foot) fasciitis (pronounced 'fashy-itis', meaning inflammation of the fascia). The plantar fascia is a thick, powerful sheet of fibrous connective tissue in the sole of the foot, complicated in design and a major preserver of the foot's longitudinal arches. It runs forwards from the heel bone until it divides into five sections called septa. Each septum further divides into two slips – a superficial one passing to the skin and a deep one that splits to enclose the flexor tendons to the toe muscles, before blending with the sole's deep ligament.

Acute plantar fasciitis causes a sharp pain under the heel when you walk or stand, extending along the inner edge of the sole. It often arises in connection with a more generalized inflammatory disease, such as gout or Reiter's disease – a form of sero-negative arthritis (*see Q 47*) that occurs in young men together with conjunctivitis and inflammation of the bladder outlet tube.

Chronic plantar fasciitis affects people aged 40–60, and usually causes less pain than the acute type. Also known as 'policeman's heel', this disorder seems to be brought on by foot-stress but can occur for no apparent reason. X-rays show either no abnormality or a bony spur projecting forwards from a prominent knobble of the heel bone. Some experts maintain that heel-bone spurs are of no significance because they are often found coincidentally in people who do not suffer from foot problems. However, evidence suggests that they can give rise to a painful inflammatory reaction in the surrounding soft tissue.

Treatment for plantar fasciitis is aimed at the accompanying inflammatory illness (if any). Pressure-relieving heel pads on an insole, together with an arch support for flat feet (if present), may be helpful, as may non-steroidal anti-inflammatory drugs (NSAIDs) or a hydrocortisone injection into the tender area. Some people claim relief from heel-bone spurs by breaking them down, by rolling a bottle or rolling pin under the sole of the foot while sitting. ●

PAGE:

~~8+7~~
8 + 9 + 10
14

BONES
(UPPER LIMBS) ?

LOWER LIMBS. [Q 69, Broken Hips Claim many Lives]
2 pages

Q 41, (Q 44 2 pages) Q 76 Q 78. CANCER OF THE BONE (MARROW
[Q 79 2 pages]

TREATMENTS

Q 82. Q 83, Q 84, Q 85, Q 88 (Q 89 (4 pages) Q 90 METHOTREXATE
                                              DRUS
[Q 95 A BOWEN THERAPY 1½ PAGES] Q 96. Aromatherapy OILS.

Bones

Introduction: Pages 6 + 7 + 8 + 9 + 0
This one →

Prevention: Q.1, Q6, Q7, Q12, Q13, Q16.
Q3   Q5
Q14, Q15, Q26, Q29, Q30, Q32.

(Q33 Arthritis) Q34,

HEAD & Neck: (Q36 2 pages) (Q40. 2 pages)

[BACTERIA REACHING THE NECK VERTEBRAE in THE
BLOODSTREAM FROM A SEPTIC SITE ELSEWHERE]

[BED-RIDDEN PATIENTS usually suffer from PNEUMONIA
Q47, Q49, Q50. [Q52 industry] Q53.

NEXT
PAGE
→

78 Our nephew, aged
four, was admitted to
hospital with a lump
about halfway down
his shinbone, and
the surgeons say
they may have to
amputate. Can they
be certain, before
doing so, that it is
cancer? And if it is,
what are his
chances?

There are several benign (non-cancerous)
swellings that affect children of your nephew's
age, but his surgical team obviously feels that the
chances of cancer are high. One possibility is Ewing's
tumour, a highly malignant form of cancer of the
bone and marrow.

Children are the usual victims. They complain of
a sore arm or leg, with pain located around the mid-
shaft region of a major long bone like the shinbone –
unlike a sarcoma, which develops at one end. A
swelling appears in the sore area, which feels firm
and warmer than the surrounding skin because
Ewing's tumour is richly supplied with blood vessels.
As the growth develops, it gradually erodes the
surrounding bone substance, and beneath the bone's
covering membrane large supplies of new bone are
formed in concentric layers (this is what causes the
'onion-peel appearance'). Both of these changes
appear on x-ray films.

Ewing's tumour is identified in a biopsy from the
singular sheets of look-alike small, round cells of
which it is composed. Radioisotope bone scanning is
also used, in which a harmless radioactive solution is
injected and the affected area is then scanned to
determine the extent of the tumour (the tumour
cells pick up the radioisotope much more readily
than the surrounding healthy tissue and are thus

easily seen). A chest X-ray may show secondary cancer deposits, for Ewing's tumour spreads rapidly, to the lungs and sometimes to other bones.

Ewing's tumour was almost always fatal, until the advent of chemotherapy, in addition to amputation – or, in some children, radiotherapy (although this is more suitable for tumours in the upper limbs). Now five-year-survival rates are recorded in more than 50 per cent of cases, so there is room for hope. ●

79 My son, who's 14, says that his knee hurts after jogging and has started to 'lock'. Does he have growing pains, or should he see a doctor?

Your son should see a doctor. 'Growing pains' is a loose term for unexplained aches and pains in the limbs and joints of children and adolescents, which need to be investigated in order to eliminate underlying disease. Your son's age, his experience of pain in the knee after running and the sudden locking suggest a condition known as osteochondritis dissecans, a disorder of convex joint surfaces in which a segment of bone below the articular cartilage loses its blood supply. It (and the cartilage) can slowly separate from the surrounding bone to form a loose body within the joint.

The cause of the disrupted blood supply is uncertain, but an inborn susceptibility to this condition probably exists. It is a disease of adolescents and young adults and, when it attacks the knee, at first causes an aching pain after exercise together with recurrent swelling due to fluid building up within the joint. After the diseased bone segment separates off, the sufferer experiences sudden locking, due to the fragment jamming between the joint surfaces during movement. The knee frequently swells and, although the range of possible movements is unaltered, the quadriceps muscle on the front of the thigh becomes wasted.

X-rays clearly show the shallow depression in a convex area within the joint, together with the bony fragment (measuring up to 2cm (¾in)) across, lying within this cavity or elsewhere within the joint. Direct inspection of the joint's interior by means of arthroscopy (see Q 82) reveals the defect in the later stages, although in the early stages the articular cartilage looks normal.

While the disease is developing the knee is supported in a crêpe bandage and strenuous activity has to be limited. Occasionally the lesion heals of its own accord; otherwise, when it is 'ripe', it should be removed, especially if it is small. If a large crater has been left, some surgeons replace the fragment and fix it with a pin, to reduce the risk of osteoarthritis occurring later on. ●

Treatments

When a bone complaint has been accurately diagnosed it is time to consider the range of possible treatments. These vary from anti-inflammatory drugs, steroids and gold injections through herbal medicines and different complementary therapies (such as chiropractic, osteopathy and acupuncture) to – in extreme cases – surgery to correct the problem. This section details the wide range of treatments on offer and their respective merits.

80 **After years of severe back pain I've been offered a spinal fusion. Might I end up in a wheelchair?**

The decision to perform a spinal fusion is generally made after consultation between orthopaedic and neurosurgical teams and a detailed discussion with the patient about the likely benefits and risks. You do not say what is wrong with your back, but the object of the operation is to relieve severe pain and/or neurological (nerve) symptoms. This entails releasing the stretched or pinched nerves, followed by fusion of the relevant spinal area, which remains permanently fixed and cannot be straightened or flexed.

Fusion for the treatment of cervical spondylosis (*see Q 36*) or spondylolisthesis uses bone grafts to bridge the vertebrae, preferably obtained from the patient (*see Q 17*). The ilium (the large wing-shaped bone forming the side of the hipbone) is the most common donor site, but the shinbone or calf bone may also be used. The technique depends upon the underlying problem as well as the surgeon's preferences. After correction of the curvature in a child with idiopathic structural scoliosis (*see Q 48*), the grafts are fitted between or alongside the spinous processes of the vertebrae (the bony knobbles you can feel under the skin of your thoracic and lumbar spine). Anterior correction and fixation by a cable screwed under tension to the vertebral bodies can be used for more severe curvatures, or for patients with abnormally shaped vertebrae.

Spinal fusion aims to improve the patient's quality of life and reduce their disability. It is, however, a major undertaking and – like all surgery – carries risks and cannot guarantee results.

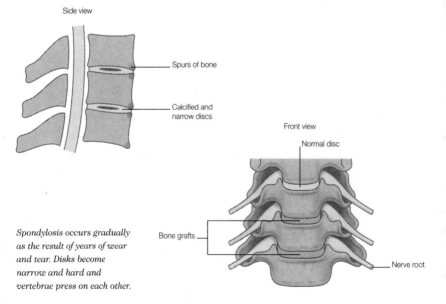

Side view

Spurs of bone

Calcified and narrow discs

Front view

Normal disc

Bone grafts

Nerve root

Spondylosis occurs gradually as the result of years of wear and tear. Disks become narrow and hard and vertebrae press on each other.

Q

81 **My husband needs an operation to remove a metal plate from his forearm. Why was it inserted in the first place?**

A surgical plate would have been inserted into your husband's forearm to 'fix' or immobilize a fracture and encourage healing. Internal fixation is used when external means, such as a splint or traction, would be inadequate; when an operation has been necessary to realign broken bones; and for limb fractures in patients with multiple injuries.

Although it is possible to fracture either forearm bone in isolation, the radius and ulna react mechanically to violence like a bundle of sticks and generally fracture together. Angulation and displacement are often marked, with a loss of contact between the upper and lower fragments in one or both bones. Rotational deformities frequently occur, making the alignment of misaligned bones without surgery impossible. Even if an acceptable position can be achieved and a plaster cast applied, the fragments often slip out of place at a later date.

For these reasons displaced fractures of the forearm bones may be realigned surgically and fixed internally, plating both bones through separate incisions. The plates are left in position for at least 21 months to lessen the risks of re-fracture. Displacement is usually slight in isolated fractures of the ulna, and a long arm plaster (for about eight weeks) is usually adequate. But if the angulation is marked, internal plating would be used.

My daughter's knee is swollen and painful after years of hard use, and she has been offered an arthroscopy. What are the risks?

Arthroscopy is a technique for obtaining direct views of a joint's interior through a fine telescope introduced into the joint via thin plastic tubing. It provides invaluable information about mechanical abnormalities, complementing that obtained from clinical assessment and x-ray.

After being given an anaesthetic, your daughter will have her knee joint filled with saline solution through a hollow needle, and the tubing and telescope will then be inserted at a suitable site – usually the inner or outer aspect of the front of the knee, depending on which compartments the surgeon wishes to inspect. By manoeuvring the telescope and using more than one entry site if necessary, the surgeon will be able to view almost the whole of the inside of the joint, with the exception of a small recess to the side and back. He will be able to gain additional information by probing the cartilages and other structures when a special probe is inserted into the joint.

Evidence of bacterial infection, tuberculosis and osteo- and rheumatoid arthritis can be gained from arthroscopy, as can signs of tears, cysts or other deformities, and injuries to the cartilages and other structures. Loose bodies within the joint, and the appearance of osteochondritis dissecans (see Q 79), may also come to light.

The risks are those associated with any minor operative procedure performed under general anaesthesia – reaction to the gases and pre-med drugs, mechanical damage to the tissues from the instruments used, and infection introduced into the knee joint despite aseptic procedures being observed. Your daughter's knee will feel painful and stiff for a week or so afterwards, but the chances of diagnosing – and, hopefully, treating – her underlying problem will be greatly increased.

83 I want my bunions removed, but the specialist warned me that it's a painful operation. Wouldn't I be prescribed painkillers?

Your doctor would certainly prescribe simple analgesia after a bunion operation, but the post-operative discomfort can be considerable, and it is important that you understand exactly what the procedure entails.

Changes preceding bunion development start with the large toe bending towards the remaining four, pushing the head of the first metatarsal inwards (*see Q 19*). The bunion (a sac) forms over the prominent metatarsal head, and the overlying skin becomes hard, red, swollen and tender. Shoe pressure aggravates the problem, and comfortable footwear becomes increasingly hard to find. Walking hurts, especially when osteoarthritis starts in the troublesome joint. Later, when the deformity is severe, the front of the foot becomes flattened and splayed, and the toes badly curled.

Bunions mainly affect women from middle age onwards, but do occur in younger women (even teenagers). The deformity usually results from persistently wearing narrow, pointed shoes – particularly high heels, which force the forefoot into the narrowest part of the shoe. You have probably already tried felt bunion pads (available from pharmacies) and wedges of plastic foam between your first and second toes to limit the deformity.

The simplest operation comprises cutting away the sac and the prominent bone without disturbing the joint. This 'displacement osteotomy' gives good results where the deformity is slight, and especially suits young patients living an energetic life. The head of the first metatarsal is removed and repositioned more naturally, eliminating the bony prominence. The toe is then kept in plaster for six weeks to ensure union of the bones. Excision arthroplasty creates a gap (a 'false joint') between the metatarsal head and the large toe's first bone, and cuts remove the bunion. This leaves a shorter, floppy large toe but relieves the pain and suits elderly people who do not walk long distances. ●

Badly fitting shoes or inherited weakness of the joints can bring about a bunion. The soft tissue at the base of the big toe becomes inflammed causing the toe to be distorted.

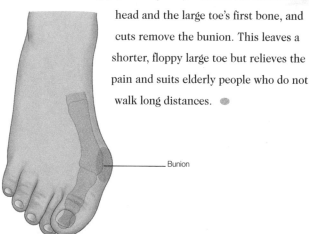

Bunion

My doctor has prescribed an anti-inflammatory drug for my painful back, to be taken only with meals. Is it likely to be dangerous?

Your medication sounds like a non-steroidal anti-inflammatory drug (NSAID). These drugs have similarities to aspirin, and they all relieve inflammation by interfering with the production of prostaglandins: short-lived, hormone-like chemicals produced in the body at specific sites, and responsible for the pain, heat, redness and swelling associated with the inflammatory reaction.

In addition to their usefulness in relieving forms of arthritis, NSAIDs are prescribed for dental pain, migraine and other headaches, period pain, some acute and chronic inflammatory conditions (such as ear and throat infections that have not responded well to antibiotics) and post-operative bone pain.

They are safe to use, provided you take them as directed and do not suffer from NSAID- or aspirin-sensitive asthma, a peptic ulcer or active bleeding anywhere in the digestive tract. Most may be prescribed under certain (carefully monitored) conditions for children, and for pregnant or nursing mothers. They should be used with caution by elderly people and anyone with a medical history of bleeding tendencies, high blood pressure, liver, kidney or heart disease. One NSAID may suit you, while others do not. Possible side-effects include gastric upset or diarrhoea, fluid retention, dizziness, buzzing in the ears, nervousness and an itchy rash.

85

After years on an anti-inflammatory drug, I started to get heartburn and my doctor changed me to a new one (celecoxib) that doesn't irritate the stomach. Will it have any side-effects?

The new anti-inflammatory celecoxib is prescribed for much the same conditions as NSAIDs (*see opposite*) and can have similar side-effects, but is generally less irritating to the digestive system. Technically, the reason for this is its ability to target and inhibit a specific enzyme named COX-2. However, celecoxib and the even newer rofecoxib still need to be taken with caution by anyone with digestive-tract problems – that is, taken with a meal and in the recommended doses. Their use needs to be monitored in people with heart, liver or kidney failure, and they interact with (among others) diuretics (water pills), aspirin, lithium, antacids and certain high-blood-pressure medications. (Note: two drugs 'interacting' does not necessarily make them incompatible; it is simply important for your doctor to know of any patent/prescribed medicines that you take regularly or occasionally, for whatever reason).

Interestingly, COX-2 inhibitors may have a role to play in cancer prevention. NSAIDs have long been known to halve the risks of developing bowel cancer, but their adverse effects on the bowel in other respects have prevented their wide use for this purpose. COX-2 inhibitors, with their better risk profile, may eventually be routinely prescribed for people with familial adenomatous polyposis (FAP): an inherited, potentially malignant condition of the large bowel. ●

86 My sister, who is 55, has rheumatoid arthritis and her doctor wants her to take steroids. What are the possible side-effects?

Rheumatologists and orthopaedic surgeons vary greatly in their use of corticosteroids (the medical name) to treat rheumatoid arthritis.

Corticosteroids (so called because they are based on natural body steroids produced in the cortex of the adrenal glands) are probably the most powerful anti-inflammatory agents known to us. They reduce the pain, heat, swelling and stiffness of arthritic joints, especially in the active phases of the disease, and convert savage pain into tolerable discomfort.

Their adverse effects are collectively referred to as Cushing's syndrome. They include tissue wasting, muscular pain and weakness, thin skin, easy bruising and excess fat laid down in the trunk, head and neck regions, producing a 'buffalo hump'. Fluid retention can lead to a full, moon-shaped face, swollen soft tissues in the legs, feet and hands, and raised blood pressure. Prolonged courses of steroids can result in an increased risk of infections and delayed wound healing, peptic ulcers, cataracts and glaucoma, while women sometimes develop unwanted body hair and find that their periods stop. There is an increased risk of developing diabetes, nerve lesions and agitation.

Despite this, corticosteroid drugs doubtless have a valuable role in the management of your sister's medical condition, and careful monitoring of her health could provide significant pain relief. ●

87 My mother's doctor injected her painful shoulder and she has had no further trouble for months. What did he use?

He will have injected your mother's shoulder with hydrocortisone, perhaps used in combination with lignocaine, a local anaesthetic. The aim of injections such as this is to provide the benefits of corticosteroid treatment (see opposite) for a painful joint or soft-tissue damage, without the disadvantages of taking a course of steroids by mouth. Most of the hydrocortisone remains in the injected area, where it relieves pain and stiffness by its anti-inflammatory action. The little that is absorbed into the body's system does only minor (if any) harm. The local anaesthetic is added to promote the injection's painkilling effects, both at the time and afterwards.

Experience and skill are needed to carry out this procedure, because it is essential to release the medication into the inflamed tissues without puncturing an artery or vein or damaging a nerve. Like most treatment it has its disadvantages, including the risk of infection (especially with repeated injections).

There is also a risk of accelerating a degenerative condition, such as certain types of arthritis, by a mechanism that is not yet fully understood; and the relief may be short-lived, although fortunately not in your mother's case. Lastly, despite the use of lignocaine, some patients experience considerable discomfort from this procedure and are unwilling to give the therapy a second chance.

Hydrocortisone injections are useful in relieving the pain of tennis elbow (*see Q 60*) and inflammation of the tendon sheath of the long biceps tendon, which causes pain and local tenderness in the groove at the top end of the upper arm bone. They can also relieve the discomfort of inflammation of the wrist tendons and the surrounding soft tissue, which is due to overuse of the hand (repetitive strain injury, or RSI) following, for instance, hours of piano practice or typing. ●

88 I've heard that gold is used to relieve rheumatoid arthritis symptoms. How can metal help a disorder such as that?

Gold has been used for decades as a 'second-line' therapy to treat rheumatoid arthritis – that is, it is prescribed for patients after 'first-line' medication, such as non-steroidal anti-inflammatory drugs (NSAIDs), has either proved unsatisfactory or has provided all the benefits that can reasonably be expected of it.

Gold is usually given as intramuscular injections of body-compatible compounds, such as aurothioglucose (gold combined with derivatives of sulphur and glucose), available in 10ml packs of an oily suspension containing 50mg in 5ml. Patients receive weekly injections, gradually increasing from a starter dose of 10mg to 50mg doses every seven days, until they have received a total of 0.8–1.0g.

Gold injections must be used with caution in patients who are suffering from arterial disease of the heart or brain; those with liver or kidney disease; and in elderly or breastfeeding patients. Regular blood tests are mandatory because gold treatment can upset the cell count and other factors in the body. Gold treatment should not be given at all to patients who are very debilitated or who suffer from severe, poorly controlled diabetes; those who are suffering from heart failure and/or moderate to severe raised blood pressure; patients with blood disorders; large bowel inflammation; eczema; or a tendency to drug allergies.

The side-effects of intramuscular gold injections may include dermatitis, inflammation of the mouth, flushing, fainting, dizziness, sweating and exhaustion as well as some kidney disorders. It is important for patients to inform specialists of any other drugs they are taking, because injected gold can enhance the effect of other medications that cause abnormalities in the blood. ●

Which natural medicines help to relieve arthritis?

Many arthritis sufferers turn to natural medicines to relieve their painful joints. Some have been disappointed with the results of orthodox drugs and treatment; others have benefited from prescribed drugs but have to stop taking them because of their side-effects; yet others – perhaps with mild to moderate symptoms – try complementary therapies before consulting their doctor, in an attempt to avoid prescription medicines. It is important to obtain a medical diagnosis for any long-standing problem, but herbal and other natural medicines produced by reputable manufacturers are safe and often effective, provided you take them as directed.

Fish oil and evening primrose oil supplements have proven benefits in treating mild to moderate arthritic pain (see Q 7). A popular remedy in recent years has been concentrated celery-seed extract, with anti-inflammatory and anti-rheumatic properties; celery extract also acts as a diuretic, combating fluid retention and helping to relieve the swelling that contributes to joint pain and stiffness. Some products combine up to 5,000mg concentrated celery oil with fish and evening primrose oil and extract of white willow bark. The original source of salicin (the forerunner of modern aspirin), white willow bark has been used worldwide for centuries to relieve the pain of inflamed joints and accompanying feverish illness. Devil's claw extract, obtained from the seed and pod of an African plant, *Harpagophytum procumbens,* has been used by native tribes to relieve the pain of arthritis for hundreds of years.

Unlike NSAIDs, herbal anti-arthritic preparations have few side-effects and are often safer to take than the pharmaceutical chemicals based upon them. ●

My sister-in-law has been diagnosed with breast cancer. She is already taking methotrexate for rheumatoid arthritis, so will this help the cancer?

The answer to your question will have to be worked out by her orthopaedic specialist in liaison with the cancer specialist responsible for her treatment. As you already know, methotrexate is used to treat both these conditions; it is also prescribed for patients with severe debilitating psoriasis (an inflammatory disease of the skin).

It works for cancer as a broad-spectrum anti-neoplastic agent, which means that it is useful in a number of malignant conditions characterized by an abnormally high multiplication of cancerous cells. It can, however, cause numerous unpleasant and/or dangerous side-effects, ranging from liver, kidney and lung disease, through certain forms of cancer and abnormalities of the bone marrow and blood, to mouth ulcers, diarrhoea, fertility changes, eye complaints, bloodclots, fever and severe skin reactions.

Methotrexate is unsuitable for any patient with bone-marrow or blood abnormalities, a severely impaired immune defence system, (most) kidney diseases or anyone who is breastfeeding; and for rheumatoid arthritis patients who have alcohol dependence or cirrhosis of the liver, peptic ulcers or ulcerative colitis.

Nevertheless, methotrexate has emerged as many specialists' first choice of DMARD (disease-modifying anti-rheumatic drug) – a concept similar to second-line medical treatment (*see Q 88*). Extensive European-American studies lasting for a period of 12 months have now shown that methotrexate produced significant clinical improvement – as well as some X-ray evidence of a slowing down of the disease process – in at least 50 per cent of patients with rheumatoid arthritis, compared with those patients who were receiving a placebo (or dummy drug substitute). ●

Q 91

I heard on the radio that bacterial toxins are being injected into patients who are suffering from joint disorders. Surely this can't be true?

I think you are referring to an injection of the toxin from the *Chlostridium botulinum* bacterium. Medical preparations of this toxin, which is known as type A, have been used for some time to treat cerebral palsy in children and facial nerve palsy. It acts on the neuromuscular junction (where a nerve meets a muscle and stimulates contractions), causing dangerous symptoms when released by the bacteria but beneficial effects when it is administered as a medical drug.

Recent US research has studied the possible benefits of this treatment in the relief of pain in the lower back: 28 patients were allocated either to the treatment group or a placebo (dummy-medicine) group; the former received 200 units of *botulinum* toxin A, and the latter normal saline injections, into the muscles running down the spine on the most painful side. All of the patients treated (whose average age was 46) had suffered from lower back pain at least six years.

Patients were advised to continue with their usual painkillers, anti-spasmodics and NSAIDs, without changing the dose. Their 'baseline' level of pain and disability (difficulty in walking, lifting, and so on) was documented at the start of the study. Professor Bahman Jabbari , head of the department of neurology at the Uniformed Services University of Health Sciences in Washington, DC, whose team conducted the study, reported that 11 out of the 14 patients in the *botulinum* group demonstrated more than 50 per cent pain relief three weeks into the study, compared with just four of the 14 patients receiving the saline injections.

Ten of the treatment group and three of the saline group demonstrated significant improvement in overall activity at eight weeks; when eight of the ten patients whose pain was significantly relieved were reviewed five to six months after treatment, all reported that the beneficial effects had worn off after about four months. No side-effects were reported, and further studies will soon be under way to establish whether repeated injections would maintain the original level of improvement. ●

Q

92 **Is chiropractic an ancient art? What is it based on, and is it safe?**

Chiropractic is a term derived from the Greek words *cheiro* and *practic,* meaning 'performed by hand'. It began in the US in the 1890s, when a magnetic healer and teacher, Dr David Palmer, restored the hearing of a man who had been deaf for 17 years by manipulating his upper-back spine. Two years later he founded the Palmer College of Chiropractic in Iowa. Chiropractic has since flourished in most developed countries, earning huge numbers of devotees and some critics.

Chiropractic is founded upon a philosophy that acknowledges the nervous system as co-ordinator of all other body structures and organs. Ill health is attributed to maladies of the central nervous system, which chiropractic manipulation seeks to rectify. Fundamental to its practice is the understanding that partial dislocation of the body's joints, or some other form of joint dysfunction, irritates the nerves and leads to abnormalities of the nervous system.

A chiropractor uses both hands to apply pressure with a twisting motion to realign the vertebrae. This helps the spine to regain some of the flexibility it looses when under strain.

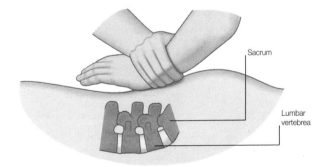

Sacrum

Lumbar vertebrea

An example is irritation of the sciatic nerve, derived from nerve roots between the fourth and fifth lumbar vertebrae and the first, second and third joints of the sacrum, due to a partial dislocation or misalignment of the vertebrae at these levels, resulting in pain in the buttock and down the leg.

A chiropractic examination aims at identifying and localizing the patient's underlying problem, and often includes nerve, muscle, skeletal and other physical tests, and possibly x-rays. The classic chiropractic treatment is the so-called 'high-velocity thrust', which consists of a quick, thrusting, painless squeeze to the patient in such a way that misaligned joints are pushed rapidly back into place. The practitioner may carry out the thrust manually or with the assistance of a spring-loaded device. Chiropractic is normally safe and effective when carried out by qualified practitioners.

93 **Since an osteopath treated me for sciatica I have been free of this problem. How does osteopathy work?**

Like chiropractic, osteopathy has been taught as an art based on its own fundamental philosophy. It proposes that many musculoskeletal (and some other) bodily disorders arise from a disturbance of fluid flow, particularly of venous blood on its return journey to the heart, and of lymph. It is greatly in demand, especially by patients who have failed to gain relief from orthodox medicine or who prefer to avoid pharmaceutical drugs and surgery.

Osteopathy was founded in Missouri in 1892 by Dr Andrew Taylor Still, a physician who had come to feel that conventional medical treatment lacked something. He concluded that mechanical problems, such as a partially dislocated vertebral joint or a minor discrepancy in leg length, could upset the venous and lymphatic return, resulting in pain and other symptoms within the neuromuscular (nerve and muscle) system, both in the affected area and at distant sites; apparently unconnected body regions were affected because of the continuity of the spinal cord and nerves, the blood and lymphatic circulation and other systems.

Another explanation stems from the holistic principle that humans and other animals are complete entities, comprising body, mind and spirit, and that a disorder in one part of the entity has repercussions elsewhere.

An osteopathic examination is aimed both at the area troubling the patient and at the rest of the body in order to identify possible causes. Sciatica, for example, may be 'caused' by a portion of intervertebral disc pressing on branches of the sciatic nerve, but reasons for this failing to heal may include disalignment in the lumbosacral spine (which, in turn, may attributed to poor posture caused by a foot or lower-limb problem). Treatment techniques include massage and manipulation, in which some practitioners include a modified form of the high-velocity thrust (see Q 92).

94 Why did physiotherapy help my son, aged 20, after his knee operation, but not my father, aged 55, with a long-standing back problem?

The successful outcome of any treatment depends on the underlying disorder, the skill of the practitioner, the patient's state of health and his ability and/or willingness to help himself. Overweight, lack of active exercise and other relevant health risks are generally more applicable to a man of your father's age than to your son's.

Physiotherapy, as we know it today, started in the early 1900s with massage techniques under a doctor's instruction. A growing repertoire of skills led hospital masseuses to adopt the professional name of physiotherapists in the 1930s and, later, the first university degree courses became available.

Physiotherapy forms an important part of non-surgical – and post-operative – orthopaedic treatment. Sometimes prescribed gratuitously as an escape route for dealing with unresponsive patients, treatment is occasionally administered without any hope of relieving a patient's symptoms. The emphasis nowadays is upon active rather than passive treatment – that is, helping the patient to help himself. This is especially beneficial in the rehabilitation of patients after injury or operation, and in cerebral palsy, stroke, nerve palsy and other illnesses. Patients need to be taught exercises that they can manage, and attend for regular treatment sessions, as well as reviews by their doctor.

Physiotherapists employ other techniques to mobilize joints, strengthen muscles and improve balance or co-ordination. Hydrotherapy is especially useful in treating rheumatoid arthritis, where the warmth and buoyancy of the water relieve muscle spasm and allow pain-free movements. Passive joint movements – especially useful after nerve injuries – help to keep the joints mobile while the patient is unable to use them himself. Electrical stimulation of the muscles can be used in conjunction with exercises, such as improving the action of the small muscles of the foot; and (after a nerve injury) to stimulate muscles to contract while awaiting the return to health of the affected nerve. ●

95 A Bowen therapy practice has started locally. What does this treatment actually do?

Bowen therapy is a system of gentle massage in which areas of muscle and connective tissue are rolled below the therapist's fingers to release obstructed energy and relieve muscular pain, and other ailments. The moves, which are gentle and non-invasive, are separated by important pauses to allow the body to benefit from a particular manoeuvre. They can be performed through light clothing and are suitable for all age groups, and the therapy is especially popular with patients who are suffering from chronic back or joint pain, and from other disorders that have not benefited from conventional treatments.

Thomas Bowen developed the therapy in Geelong, Victoria, in Australia, some three decades ago, and in 1974 he invited two other health practitioners, Oswald Rentsch and his wife Elaine, to study it with him. Under Bowen's guidance, the Rentschs observed and documented his technique, providing the therapy with a structured form while preserving its procedures and tenets. They thus founded what became known worldwide as Bowen therapy.

Bowtech – the Bowen technique, as it has been known since 1987 – is available in treatments lasting from a few minutes to over an hour, depending upon the patient's needs and responses. Based upon the holistic principle of harnessing the body's own self-healing powers (*see Q 92*), Bowen therapy stimulates energy flow in affected areas and promotes healthy, deep relaxation lasting for hours or days afterwards. Results vary from immediate relief following a single treatment to no response after a series, but Bowtech is sufficiently successful to claim worldwide recognition and to be taught in Australia, New Zealand, the UK, Europe and the US.

Studies have shown that athletes have a consistently higher performance rate and superb injury recovery after they have received Bowtech, which is also used to treat neck and back pain, repetitive strain injury (RSI), migraine, menstrual problems, arthritis and other joint disorders and injuries, as well as asthma, sinusitis and bronchial (breathing) difficulties. ●

Some natural therapists combine aromatherapy oils with massage treatment. Do these do any good?

Aromatherapy oils can be highly effective in relieving aching joints and other skeletal problems, provided they are used with care. This means selecting only pure, chemical-free essential oils and following the package directions or the advice of a doctor or qualified complementary practitioner. They should not be taken by mouth and, because they are potent and volatile when undiluted, they are blended with a 'carrier' oil when used for massage, to ensure their safe passage through the skin and into the bloodstream.

Sweet almond oil, light and emollient, is the ideal base for a general massage. Apricot kernel oil is rich in vitamins A and E, and ideal for massaging the neck and facial muscles. Jojoba, the most luxurious carrier oil, is also excellent for delicate skin areas and for treating the upper spine, neck and scalp.

Essence of arnica *(Arnica montana)* is used for treating sporting injuries, including bruises, strains, sprains and inflamed, painful joints. It quickly clears the discoloration of bruises and soothes torn, damaged ligaments, tendons and muscles. Essence of hypericum *(Hypericum perforatum,* St John's wort) produces a calming, soothing infusion for an overall body massage following an injury such as a fracture or sprain. Its local analgesic and antiseptic actions promote healing of cuts, scratches and other abrasions.

Lavender essence is also soothing, with pain-quelling properties; lemongrass has a toning effect; and ginger is a warming, soothing painkiller. While all these essential oils (and others) make healing additions to massage oils, you can also add a few drops to a basin of water and soak the affected body area. Many people inhale essential oils from a burner, heated electrically or by means of a night light. And a few drops of aromatherapy oil on a handkerchief under your pillow allows your whole system to benefit from the healing properties of essential oils while you sleep.

97 Does acupuncture relieve painful joint conditions? And how does the medical profession view this natural therapy?

To answer your second question first, the medical profession is divided on the merits of acupuncture. Although one in six Australian doctors practises it, controversy continues over whether it actually works.

Acupuncture can bring significant relief from upper and lower back disorders; neck stiffness; migraine and other headaches; arthritic pain; sciatica; and slowly healing bone, tendon, joint and ligament injuries. Numerous patients claim it as the one therapy to help when other treatments have failed. Apart from occasionally causing such deep relaxation that tiredness and lethargy persist for a day or two after treatment, it has few side-effects. Many people, in fact, report an increase in energy and a sensation of balanced calm, in addition to relief from their ailment. Explanations for its actions differ in Western and Chinese points of view.

Western (orthodox) doctors claim that acupuncture has a largely placebo effect – that is, it works on the expectation of a beneficial effect – but this does not explain how acupuncture practised by veterinary surgeons relieves an animal's symptoms. Doctors also attribute its success to the production of pain-relieving endorphins by the body, in response to stimulation of the acupuncture points. This does not fully explain how it relieves such disparate disorders as alcohol dependence, skin rashes, allergies, slowly healing fractures and low back pain.

Chinese medicine is based on the concept of Ch'i (the Life Force), which in health flows evenly through long lines of energy channels (meridians) below the skin. Ill health comes about when one or several meridians become blocked, obstructing the flow of Ch'i; causes include stress, toxins, nutritional deficiencies and an imbalance between the forces of nature manifest in all living organisms, Yin and Yang.

Acupuncture needles are round ended thus allowing them to part the skin rather than draw blood.

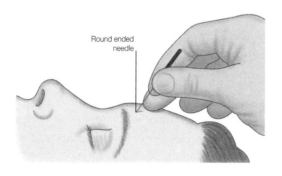

Round ended needle

The flow of Ch'i is restored (and symptoms relieved) by stimulating the acupuncture points along appropriate meridians with needles (or, now, electronically or by laser).

**What does
naturopathy do?
Could it help my
husband's backache,
which specialists
say he must learn
to live with?**

Naturopathy is worth trying for your husband's
backache. Naturopathic practitioners work
holistically on the principle that we are tripartite
combinations of body, mind and spirit. They
interpret ailments as imbalances between these
three elements, and aim to restore well being
through natural methods. They are also eclectic,
using diet, nutritional supplements, hydrotherapy,
medical herbalism and acupuncture as necessary
(sometimes through referral to other therapists) to
restore healthy function.

Obesity aggravates backache, and naturopaths
encourage healthy eating, which in turn encourages
weight loss. This eliminates fat-ridden junk foods
and high-fat, high-sugar processed dishes, and
concentrates on fibre-rich cereals and pastas, salads
of pulses, lentils and grains, and a wide range of raw
foods (vegetables and fruit), including freshly
squeezed juices, sprouts, seeds and nuts. Foods rich
is the amino acid L-tryptophan (turkey, beef, lamb
and nuts) can help to ease muscular pain by
promoting the production of serotonin. This natural
brain chemical can boost the spirits and raise the
pain threshold, reducing pain perception.

Many naturopathic practitioners also use allergy
testing to 'fine-tune' dietary recommendations to a
client's needs. Your husband may also be advised to

avoid certain foods that aggravate joint pain in some sufferers, such as citrus fruit, tomatoes and red meat. His therapist may also prescribe a multivitamin and mineral supplement to ensure that baseline nutritional requirements are met, plus high-potency vitamin B-complex in order to combat stress and tension (potent causes of muscular pain), and vitamin C and other antioxidants to boost the immune system.

At its simplest hydrotherapy consists of bathing at certain temperatures with, perhaps, the addition of aromatherapy essences or mineral salts to soothe and revive tired back muscles. Colonic irrigation (washing impurities out of the large bowel) is sometimes recommended, together with exercise, massage, manipulation and daily relaxation. ●

99 **Both my sons, aged 11 and 15, have flat feet, and I have heard that this can affect them physically and emotionally. Is an operation the only answer?**

Your sons are most unlikely to need an operation to correct their flat feet. Babies are born with flat feet, the condition is common in pre-school children and it affects ten per cent of teenagers. Children have flat feet because their joints are loose and flexible, allowing the arch to mould to a flattened shape when they are standing, and generally flat-footedness is nothing to worry about.

When a child starts to walk he places his feet widely apart and they roll at his ankles. As he grows, his ankle muscles strengthen, so that his feet gradually take shape. About 80 per cent of children develop an inner foot arch by the age of six, and a recent Australian study has cast doubt on whether flat-footed children need orthotics (rehabilitation through supportive devices) to improve their overall movement skills or general emotional well being.

Researchers reported that flat-footed children can perform muscular and movement skills as well as – or better than – their high-arched peers; and that their self-esteem was on a par with that of other children. But they reported that the jury remained 'well and truly out' on whether flat-footed children might need orthotic foot supports to overcome any pain associated with undeveloped longitudinal foot arches. If a flat-footed child shows no untoward symptoms, there seems to be no need for correction.

Flat feet are hereditary and may, in rare instances, be stiff and uncomfortable. Orthotics generally do not help, and special shoes are seldom needed. Footwear for a flat-footed child should, however, be comfortable, flexible and protective. It should allow freedom of movement and space for the foot to grow. Boots offer no advantages over shoes and, if the child's shoes become overly worn on the inner side, then shoes with a stiffer heel and an inbuilt arch support may help. ●

I have been told to practise stretch exercises before going for a daily aerobic walk, but my sports-mad son tells me that stretching is falling out of favour. Please advise me – I'm confused!

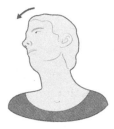

Tip head back

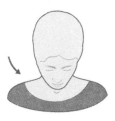

Slowly roll head towards the chest

Gentle, carefully controlled exercises rolling the head can help regain some of the loss of movement which can occur as the result of problems in the back and neck.

Stretch exercises are still prescribed beneficially for certain spinal and limb disorders, including postural problems and as a means of strengthening the muscles controlling the hip and knee, shoulder and elbow joints. They have also been a recognized part of the preliminary warm-up in athletics and fitness training for decades. The rationale for this sort of stretching is that it lengthens muscles and improves flexibility, thus preventing muscle tears and strains. However, a 1997 study of 1,538 Australian army recruits, reported in the February 2000 issue of the *American College of Sports Medicine Journal,* found that pre-exercise stretching did not in fact reduce injuries to the lower limb.

This finding resulted in the removal of stretching from the pre-exercise routine of army recruits, who now spend their warm-up time doing less demanding forms of the activities they are about to pursue during training. Since 1997 injury rates have fallen from 33 to 10 per cent, and while other measures

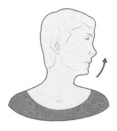

Gently roll head to the left

were introduced to help prevent injuries, lack of stretching has had no adverse effects. In fact, athletes who do not 'stretch' seem less likely to suffer joint, tendon and

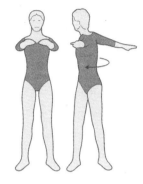

muscle damage. Concentrating on warm-up stretches can result in sportspeople neglecting more important injury-prevention measures, such as building up fitness, improving technique and carrying out appropriate light activities prior to training.

Part of the problem is that athletes concentrating on warm-up stretching extend their muscles to a length that the actual sport never demands. As Dr Chris Bradshaw, the sports-physician manager of the Australian Olympics athletics team, commented:, 'What's the point of stretching your hamstrings so that you can place your palms flat on the floor, if you never have to do that during a game?' Of therapeutic stretching, though, he comments, 'Stretching is still important if you suffer from reduced flexibility due to a previous injury or genetic (i.e. birth) predisposition.' It is also recommended for people with stiff, painful lower backs and with poor flexibility of the muscles controlling the buttocks, and hipbone area.

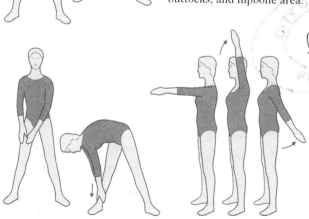

[139]

Useful Information

FURTHER READING

ANDERSON, FREEDOLPH, *Build Bone Health: Prevent and Treat Osteoporosis*, Impakt Communications, 1999

HOFFMAN, DAVID, *Healthy Bones and Joints – A Natural Approach*, Newleaf, 2001

CHAITOW, LEON, *Arthritis*, Thorsons, 1998

DEPARTMENT OF HEALTH, *Nutrition and Bone Health*, The Stationery Office, 1998

LIOC, BUM, *Back and Neck Pain: The Facts*, Oxford University Press, 1999

MELZACK, RONALD and WALL, PATRICK, *The Challenge of Pain* (Revised Edition), Penguin Books, 1996

SMITH, TONY (ED.), *BMA Family Doctor Series: Osteoporosis*, Dorling Kindersley, 1999,

THEODOSAKIS, JASON, ET AL., *The Arthritis Cure*, Century, 1997

SOBEL, DAVA AND KLEIN, ARTHUR C., *Arthritis: The Complete Guide to Relief using Methods that Really Work*, Constable, 1998

WALL, PATRICK, *Pain: The Science of Suffering*, Weidenfeld and Nicolson, 2000

USEFUL ADDRESSES

Arthritis Care
18 Stephenson Way
London NW1 2HD
tel: 020 7380 6500

The Arthritis Foundation of Ireland
1 Clan William Square
Grand Canal Quay
Dublin 2, Ireland
tel: 01 661 8188
website:
http://www.arthritis-foundation.com

British Acupuncture Council
Park House
206–208 Latimer Road
London W10 6RE
tel: 020 87350400

British Chiropractic Association
Blagrave House, Blagrave Street,
Reading RG21 1QB
tel: 0118 950 5950

British School of Osteopathy
275 Borough High Street
London SE1 1JE
tel: 020 7407 0222

The Chartered Society of
Physiotherapy
14 Bedford Row, London WC1R 4ED
tel: 020 7306 6663/4/5

The Society of Teachers of the
Alexander Technique
20 London House, 266 Fulham Road
London SW10 9EL
tel: 020 7351 0828
e-mail: enquiries@stat.org.uk

Chiropractor's Association of
Australia (National) Ltd
Suite 4, 148 Station Road
Penrith, NSW 2750
tel: 02 4731 8011
website:
http://www.caa.com.au

WEBSITES

BackCare, the National Organization
for Healthy Backs
http://www.backpain.org

Low back pain and sciatica
http://www.voiceoftheinjured.com/
a-si-back-spine-pain-sciatica-diagnosis-
treatment.html

National Center for Complementary
and Alternative Medicine
http://www.nccam.nih.gov/nccam/fcp/
factsheets/acupuncture/acupuncture.htm

Neck pain
http://www.wadhurst-physio.co.uk/
neck%20pain.htm

Scoliosis, osteoporosis, Paget's disease
http@//yourhealth.queens.org/Health
Topics/

Chiropractic Association of Ireland
http://www.chiropractic.ie

The Arthritis Webpages of drdoc on-line
http://www.arthritis.co.za

Index

misalignment, 16
multiple, 34, 112
orbit, 60
rib, 65
scaphoid, 92
stress, 19, 97, 98
transverse, 83, 84
undiagnosed, 15
wedge-compression, 64
Fragile bone disease, 34-5
Funny bone, *see ulna*

G

Ganglia, 89-90
Gangrene, 55
Gold injections, 48, 120, 121
Gout, 26, 45, 46, 106

H

Hand, 90, 91, 92
Hip
bone, 41, 43, 66, 73, 95
broken, 94-5
joint, 14, 24, 95, 99
pain, 99, 100
pregnancy, 13
Hormonal replacement
therapy (HRT), 39
'Housemaid's knee', 101, 102
Human growth hormones
(HGH), 42
Human skeleton, 7, 22
Humerus (upper arm), 15,
20
Hydrocortisone injections,
48, 75, 83, 106, 119-20
Hydrotherapy, 130, 136

I

Immune system, 48
Inflammation, 18, 46, 47,
53, 56, 101

J

Joint
ball and socket, 79
capsule, 77, 78, 80, 86,
87, 90, 91
deformity, 41
degenerative changes, 50
haemophilia damage, 26
intervertebral, 68, 70,
128
replacement, 41
sacro-coccygygial, 75
sacro-iliac, 66, 74

K

Knee
cap, 22, 23, 100, 101
joint, 44, 47, 101, 102
pain, 108,
swelling, 109
Kyphosis (spinal curve), 24,
68

L

Ligaments, 22-3, 31-2, 35,
61, 66, 80, 87, 96, 105
Lordosis (exaggerated
hollow back), 24, 36, 241
Lower back pain, 27, 66,
71, 74, 124, 125

M

Manipulation, 53, 74, 75,
77
Membranes, 20, 49, 59
Meningitis, 37
Menopause, 40, 88
Muscle
deltoid, 79, 85
fatigue, 97
flexor, 87
intercostal, 32, 65
spasm, 47
strain, 19

N

Natural medicines, 121-2
Naturopathy, 135-6
Neck, 32, 52, 53, 54, 55,
56, 61, 66
Nerves, 14, 90
damage, 57
endings, 51, 82
Nodules (tophi), 45

O

Obesity, 26, 50, 135
Oesteochondroma (benign
bone tumour), 44
Orthotic brace, 24, 67
Osteoarthritis, *see arthritis*
Osteochondritis dissecans,
108, 113
Osteopathy, 127-8
Osteoporosis (brittle bone
disease), 7, 16, 28, 39,
40, 43, 57, 58, 84, 94
Osteosarcoma, 30

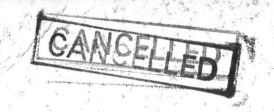